To all of my wonderful patients,
who taught me more than I taught them.

apple, carrot, kale, ginger, beets
liver tonic

stop aging, start living

stop aging, start living

THE REVOLUTIONARY 2-WEEK PH DIET
THAT ERASES WRINKLES, BEAUTIFIES SKIN,
AND MAKES YOU FEEL FANTASTIC

JEANNETTE GRAF, M.D.
with alisa bowman

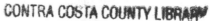

CROWN PUBLISHERS
new york

Copyright © 2007 by Jeannette Graf, M.D.

All rights reserved.
Published in the United States by Crown Publishers, an imprint of the Crown Publishing Group, a division of Random House, Inc., New York.
www.crownpublishing.com

Crown is a trademark and the Crown colophon is a registered trademark of Random House, Inc.

Library of Congress Cataloging-in-Publication Data

Graf, Jeannette.
Stop aging, start living : the revolutionary 2-week pH diet that erases wrinkles, beautifies skin, and makes you feel fantastic / by Jeannette Graf with Alisa Bowman.—1st ed.
p. cm.
Includes bibliographical references and index.
1. Nutrition.   2. Acid-base imbalances—Diet therapy.   3. Acid-base equilibrium.
4. Skin—Care and hygiene.   5. Women—Health and hygiene.   6. Self-care, Health.
I. Bowman, Alisa.   II. Title.
RA784.G688 2007
646.7'26—dc22   2007013258

ISBN 978-0-307-38236-8

Printed in the United States of America

Design by Debbie Glasserman

10 9 8 7 6 5 4 3 2 1

First Edition

acknowledgments

To Todd Shuster, Rachel Sussman, Sandra Shagat, and the rest of the team at Zachary Shuster Harmsworth Literary for believing in this project from its infancy.

To Heather Jackson for her always useful guidance and motivating enthusiasm. Every author should have such a talented editor. You're a complete joy. We're also grateful to Mary Choteborsky, Donna Passannante, Christine Aronson, Tina Constable, Kristin Kiser, Selina Cicogna, and the rest of the team at Crown for their support, direction, and expertise.

To Karen Oliver, of Karen Oliver and Associates, for getting the word out to beauty editors across the country about the importance of pH for beautiful skin.

To Greg Thompson, executive chef at Morton's The Steakhouse in South Park, Charlotte, North Carolina, for doing the impossible: creating the delicious, quick, and easy alkalinizing recipes included in this book. Thanks to you, we now know how to cook kale that tastes as good as it is good for us.

To New York City nutritionist Leslie Dantchik, M.S., for overseeing the menu plan, serving as an expert reviewer for much of the book's nutrition content, and lending a few of your own fabulous recipes to the project. Thanks for always going the extra mile and never complaining, no matter how insane our requests.

To Georgene Grella, the aesthetician who works with me, and Mary McGuire, who runs americanyogini.com. They were kind enough to share their personal skin care recipes with me.

To Dr. Robert Bienkowski, without whose friendship and guidance none of this would have been possible.

To Dr. Hynda Kleinman, a great mentor and friend who taught me cell biology and treated me as family while I was at the National Institutes of Health.

To Dr. George R. Martin, my laboratory chief at the National Institutes of Health, whose brilliance, scientific integrity, and friendship have had an enormous and everlasting impact on my career.

To my husband, Bennett, for tolerating my late-night interviews and research missions.

To my wonderful children, Jordan and Michelle, the precious loves of my life. Thank you for inspiring me and reminding me to laugh.

To my dear parents, Edmund and Malvina Graf, who survived the unthinkable to come to America so that I could have a life filled with freedom and the choice to live my dreams.

To my co-author, Alisa Bowman, for not only putting my ideas into words but also enthusiastically living the Stop Aging, Start Living program.

—JEANNETTE GRAF, M.D.

To my husband, Mark, for his endless support. On those rare occasions when I forget why I ever became a writer in the first place, you always remember why and gently tell me so.

To my beautiful, joy-filled, precious daughter, Kaarina. You make life worth living. You inspire my every word.

To my parents, Don and Marilyn, for always believing in me.

To my high school journalism teacher, Miss Hayden, for giving me a lifelong love of words.

To my co-author, Jeannette Graf, M.D., for making me younger inside and out. You're a wonderful friend. You make my job way too fun.

—ALISA BOWMAN

contents

stop aging, start living

introduction

You're in the bookstore or shopping online and you're considering buying this book. You picked it up because something bothers you about the way you look. You may not be fully aware of what it is. You just know that you are not particularly fond of mirrors these days.

So you're holding this book and a part of your brain is telling you, "Buy it! It's the answer. It will make me young again! I'll erase five years overnight!" Another part of your brain is telling you, "This is garbage. There's no way anything can help me. I need plastic surgery."

Which thought will you listen to? I hope you choose the first over the second. That's the thought I chose to listen to when I first met Dr. Jeannette Graf, and she did not disappoint. Her program works. You will look younger overnight and transformed in two weeks. Your skin will be brighter, smoother, and softer than it has been in years. You will feel dramatically younger and happier, too. I know, because I do.

Her program is based on science, science that is perfectly valid but not well known outside the field of medicine. It uses specific eating prescriptions, supplements, and lifestyle suggestions to slow cellular aging everywhere inside the body—including in the cells that make up the skin. By alkalinizing cellular fluids, improving digestion, and increasing the production and effectiveness of specific brain chemicals, the program creates a glow and radiance that no amount of money can buy. Dr. Graf's program also involves the use of effective yet affordable skin care products that brighten, soften, smooth, and beautify the skin from the outside in.

The first time I spoke with Dr. Graf, I was struggling to keep my life together. I was a working mom of an eight-month-old daughter (now she's two and a half). I was married to a man who had recently started a new business and was working twelve-hour days, seven days a week (now he occasionally takes a day off, and works ten-hour days instead). I was nursing, and my daughter had me up every two hours at night. She was also frequently sick and extremely distrustful of all other adults. If someone else tried to hold her so I could relax, she screamed.

Needless to say, I felt dreadful and looked the same. My hair was falling out. My eyes were ringed with dark circles. My complexion was pale and flaky. My cheeks were mottled with uneven brownish splotches known as chloasma, or the "mask of pregnancy." I had crow's feet and frown lines. I spent my days yearning for coffee and fantasizing about sleep. I was emotionally sour, angry, depressed— you name it. I wasn't myself. Pregnancy, childbirth, and motherhood had aged me five years, if not ten.

So that was me, a woman barely alive, on one end of a landline. On the other end was Jeannette, the Energizer Bunny. I could tell by the sound and strength of her voice that Jeannette was the type of person who kept going and going—and loved it. In her voice I heard happiness. I heard energy. I heard fun, joy, and laughter. I heard the sound of the person I wanted to become.

As we spoke, Jeannette described the results her patients experienced. I'll admit, after spending more than twelve years in the health-writing business, I was more than a little skeptical when she told me that patients saw immediate results—as in *overnight immediate results*. I also wasn't so sure of the theory. I had heard of the importance of body pH for overall health. I wasn't so sure it affected skin health.

Yet I wanted what Jeannette had. Something told me to trust her. "Sign me up," I told her. We were a perfect book-writing match.

Jeannette had the information I needed to turn my skin and my life around. I had the skills she needed to put her program on paper.

I soon learned that I was doing nearly everything wrong. I washed my face with a detergent-based soap, which stripped my already dry skin of moisture. I didn't use moisturizer, rarely wore sunscreen, and at times didn't bother to wash my face after exercise or before bed. All bad, but easily remedied with a trip to the store to purchase a cleanser, moisturizer, and other products designed for my specific skin type.

My lifestyle needed some changing, too. I got little sleep (a problem I couldn't easily remedy at the time) and set off my stress response about once every five minutes. Over a period of months, with Jeannette's coaxing, I began taking more time for myself. I stopped feeling guilty about napping when I was tired, cut back on my work commitments, and began shielding myself from people who generally annoyed me. I added joy and fun back into my life, making time to go to book group (something I loved but had stopped after my baby was born), to take a stress reduction class, and to run with my favorite running partner (someone who—without fail— always made me smile).

I incorporated other changes as well. I ate more vegetables and less meat and sugar. I drank more water and took Jeannette's supplements religiously. I chewed my food more thoroughly. I laughed more—a lot more.

Her program changed my life, my looks, and my energy. That's why I know it can change yours as well. These days when I catch my reflection in a mirror, I sometimes actually turn up the light to get a better look. That's how much I like what I see! My face is brighter. My skin is softer—so soft that I'll occasionally brush it with my fingertips in wonder. My eyes look alive. My lines are less noticeable.

Interestingly, my cholesterol, which had been over 200 since my early twenties, came down to 175 with this program. The change was so dramatic that I asked my doctor if the lab might have given me someone else's results! I'm also more joyful and happy. Before I did this program, it was a struggle for me to smile. It felt forced. Now I smile naturally. I'm happy on the inside, and it shows on the outside. I'm also a better mother and wife. I've put Jeannette's fun prescription to good use, and it has provided me with plenty of moments to laugh hysterically with my daughter as we jump up and down to songs and just generally act silly. I have the energy for it, too.

You may be wondering what you have to do to experience such wonderful results. The program involves four key prescriptions.

The Nutrition Prescription. You'll focus most of your food choices on Jeannette's eleven alkalinizing Age Stoppers (dark leafy greens, vegetables, filtered water, lemons and limes, garlic and onions, spices, fruit, nuts and seeds, olive oil, sea salt, and specific whole grains) and try to minimize the five acid-producing Age Accelerators (sugar, processed carbohydrates, alcohol, colas, coffee, and animal protein). Using her 3-to-1 alkalinizing formula, you can continue to eat the acid-producing foods you love by balancing them with more alkaline options.

The Supplement Prescription. Each morning you'll drink a sweet but powerfully effective Alkalinizing Cocktail that contains greens powder and fiber. You'll also take an alkalinizing mineral supplement with calcium and a probiotic supplement to improve digestion.

The Lifestyle Prescription. Through laughter (watching funny movies), joy (doing something every week that exhilarates you), and calm (deep breathing, vegging out, etc.), you'll rev up brain chemicals that produce joy, happiness, serenity, and an overall sense of well-being. Your skin will glow as a result.

The Skin Care Prescription. By using a cleanser, moisturizer, sunblock, eye cream, and makeup suitable for your age, skin type, and skin needs, you'll reduce the appearance of wrinkles and plump up your skin. The products work, and they're affordable and easy for even the least knowledgeable skin care consumer (read: me) to find. You won't go broke on this program.

Jeannette has worked with enough patients over the years to know that there can sometimes be a disconnect between knowing what to do for your skin and actually doing it. To help you put the program into practice, she's included quick and easy alkalinizing recipes, especially recipes for the greens that are so important to skin health. She's also included three plan options, depending on your personal level of motivation.

If you are really motivated and able to make a lot of changes at once, you can do the 24-Hour Kick-Start Plan, which includes a day of intense but effective Stop Aging activities. Or you can follow the 2-Week Plan, which provides daily menus, recipes, and checklists to help you stay on track.

Or you can do what I did, and incorporate a few Stop Aging strategies into your life as they suit you. It's a slower approach and the results are not as dramatic, but they are impressive nonetheless. No matter how you tackle the program, I can tell you that you won't be sorry. This plan works. Stop aging right now. Keep reading to learn how.

part 1

How do you stop aging? You do so one cell at a time. The health of your entire body and the health of your skin are connected in at least three important ways.

The pH connection. The enzymes, proteins, peptides, and cells that form your skin and body all function best when the fluid that surrounds them remains at a specific pH. Allow that pH to drop too low—usually through an acid-producing diet—and cells do not function effectively.

The digestion connection. Your skin needs specific nutrients and can get these nutrients only if your intestines absorb them from the food you eat. Poor digestion—usually caused either by a low-fiber diet or by an imbalance of gut bacteria—can prevent certain nutrients from getting absorbed. It also may allow harmful substances to gain entry to the bloodstream, and eventually to the cells in the skin.

The joy connection. Nerves and chemicals called neuropeptides link your skin to your brain. For this reason, the health of the neurons and peptides in your brain greatly affects your skin. This is why positive emotions can make your skin glow and why negative emotions (guilt, sadness, depression) lead to an ashen appearance. Stress is particularly harsh on your skin, triggering rashes and acne, accelerating the formation and growth of skin cancer, and aggravating dryness and dullness.

In Part One of this book, I explain all of these connections in a simple, straightforward way so that you can understand how the Stop Aging, Start Living Plan works. I invite you to accompany me on an eye-opening journey to discover how improving pH, brain function, and digestion will help you to stop aging.

1

stop aging—one cell at a time

Not long ago, Susan, a tall fair-skinned lawyer in her late forties, walked into my office and asked me to help her look younger. "I want to look better. I don't know what's wrong. I think I'm doing everything right, but my skin just doesn't look great," she told me.

Like so many patients, Susan had done just about everything before seeking my advice. She had willingly undergone numerous cosmetic procedures with various doctors and aesthetic specialists, her face alternately lasered, lifted, injected with Botox, and filled with collagen. Although these procedures had erased any hint of a wrinkle, they hadn't given Susan the youthful appearance she sought. Susan wanted radiance and smoothness, yet her skin was dull, dry, and pale.

I invited Susan to sit down with me for a few minutes and asked her about her diet, lifestyle, and skin care practices. She told me she had spent the past few months on a low-carbohydrate diet, which meant that most days she ate from two food groups: chicken breast and Diet Coke. Each morning, she took a long, hot shower. "It's the only way I can wake up," she told me. After a stressful day at work, she hit the gym, running on the treadmill, taking kick-boxing classes, and making her way around the Nautilus circuit. She then showered, dressed, and drove home, where, after more chicken and

Diet Coke, she plopped down in front of the TV, watching gory crime dramas, until she finally dragged herself to bed.

I asked Susan how she felt. She told me that she felt tired a lot of the time. She frequently suffered from gas and bloating. She had trouble sleeping at night.

"What do you do for fun?" I asked.

"What do you mean?" she replied. I learned that Susan's days were filled with work, volunteer work, and family responsibilities. She didn't have time for "fun."

I nodded. Her symptoms, habits, and lifestyle sounded so familiar, I hardly needed to make notes in her chart. "I would like to try something with you," I told her.

I pulled a pH strip from a supply cabinet and asked Susan to place it on her tongue. After a few seconds, I removed the strip. Sure enough, Susan's saliva pH of 6.0 indicated to me that the pH levels of the fluids in her body were probably far too acidic for the optimal functioning of the cells in her skin.

That's when I knew there was little I could do with fillers, peels, and other office procedures to create the vibrancy, radiance, and smoothness Susan sought. For these results, Susan would have to make some dietary and lifestyle changes. Susan's diet was causing acids to build up in her organs, tissues, and cells—including the important cells in the inner layer of her skin. Her diet also led to poor digestion, which prevented important nutrients from getting to her skin. Her excessive showering was stripping the outer layer of her skin of moisture, making it appear thin and brittle. Her stressful lifestyle only magnified her problems.

As I explained all of this to Susan, I mixed an Alkalinizing Cocktail. I stirred a packet of greens powder into a glass of water, along with a scoop of fiber and spirulina (blue-green algae).

"You want me to drink that?" Susan asked.

I laughed. "You've endured knives and needles trying to get the skin of your dreams," I reminded her. "I know this doesn't look appetizing, but it actually tastes sweet. More important, it's full of fiber, antioxidants, plant nutrients, and enzymes. One glass provides the body with the equivalent nutrition of ten servings of organic fruits and vegetables."

Susan finished the drink easily while I described the principles of my simple skin program. After a few minutes, I asked Susan to look in the mirror. Her skin and eyes had begun to brighten. Although Susan had arrived at my office tired and stressed—this doctor visit just one more task in her busy day—her body responded instantly when we gave it what it needed. She was pleasantly surprised. I gave Susan the ingredients for the Alkalinizing Cocktail so she could make it at home. I also gave her a few skin care products to use each morning and night. Finally, I encouraged her to do something really fun that night.

The following morning, as soon as I walked into the office, Susan was on the phone. "Everyone tells me that I look radiant, that my eyes are brighter," she said. "I have more energy, too!" That day Susan embarked on my comprehensive 2-Week Plan, and she's been referring friends and colleagues to me ever since.

A Few Simple Principles Backed by Science

If you have doubts that a strange-looking drink, some moisturizer, and a little bit of fun can produce *any* results, not to mention *overnight* results, please rest assured that I am a board-certified physician who makes only nutritional, lifestyle, and skin care recommendations that are backed by good science. I began my career in the laboratories of the National Institutes of Health (NIH), so I am familiar with the scientific method and have relied on it, along with scores of reputable studies, to guide and support my advice. While at the NIH, I was a research scientist. I spent my days peering into microscopes to see skin cells up close. My studies, done at the NIH and elsewhere, have appeared in a number of prestigious scientific journals such as *Cell, Science,* the *Journal of Cell Biology,* the *Proceedings of the National Academy of Sciences,* and *Biochemistry.* I even won an Outstanding Achievement Award for one of my discoveries. So please understand that I do know the difference between true science and marketing-driven quackery. All of my recommendations are based on research.

I've also worked with thousands of patients during my more than fifteen years in private practice. I didn't create the plan you'll find in this book overnight. It came to me after treating patient after patient who, on the surface, seemed to be doing everything right. These patients had excellent cosmetic results with various topical treatments that I prescribed or formulated, as well as with Botox, collagen, and Restylane, but they didn't look great. They were missing vibrancy and luster.

I also noticed that some other patients who had not undergone as many procedures actually looked more alive and vibrant. I wanted to know what these naturally younger-looking patients were doing that my other patients were not, so I began asking questions about their diet, lifestyle, and skin care habits.

I also began an intense study of available skin care research. I examined more than one hundred years of studies, some of them Nobel Prize–winning. Each study provided a nugget of information that I then tested on my patients and on myself.

From my patients and my own trial and error, I've learned many important lessons. Not only have I learned what skin care and lifestyle practices are *most* important for skin health, I've also learned which practices everyday folks such as yourself will likely adopt, and which ones you'll find too cumbersome to deal with. For instance, eating ten servings daily of organic, raw vegetables is undoubtedly good for your skin. Yet most people just can't and won't make such a huge lifestyle change. Coffee isn't the greatest for your skin. Will you give it up if you are a die-hard espresso fan? I doubt it. I certainly haven't.

I realized that my patients needed a realistic way to *balance* their bad habits with realistic good habits. During the past few years, my discoveries gelled into a specific, realistic, and effective program, the one you will find in this book. It works. I know, because I've seen it work for every single patient who has tried it.

It has also worked for me. I'm a working mom with two teenage kids and an aging father who is in and out of the hospital. I travel. I have a busy private practice. I consult with cosmetic companies. I write books. Is it stressful? You bet! Do I have lots of time to grow organic vegetables in my backyard, chop and dice, or follow a raw food diet? Not if my life depended on it! I'm busy. I focus on lifestyle changes that provide me with the maximum benefit for my time.

I also love coffee and red wine—both of which are no-no's when it comes to beautiful skin (you'll soon learn why). I also frequently get too little sleep. These are all facts of my life, yet this program has worked for *me*. That's why I'm convinced it will work for *you*.

Will you have to make some changes in order to stop aging and start living? Of course, but those changes will be *realistic* changes. This program doesn't ask you to do anything that I personally couldn't do myself. If I can sustain this lifestyle, so can you. If you don't believe me, believe the stories of the many patients you'll read about throughout the pages of this book. They, too, had real lives with real problems and hard-to-part-with bad habits. Yet they were able to stop aging and start living. You can, too.

I call this the Stop Aging, Start Living Plan because that's what it does. Not only does this program help you to look more youthful on the outside, it also slows the aging of every cell in your body *on the inside*. As a result, you not only appear younger, you grow younger. Your cholesterol level, blood pressure, and blood sugar will drop. Digestion will improve, so you will no longer suffer from gas, bloating, or constipation. Headaches will diminish. You may even find that your cravings for unhealthful foods diminishes, and continue to diminish the longer you follow this plan. Today you may not be able to get by without your cigarettes, sugary treats, or soft drinks, but these foods and substances will eventually lose their appeal.

Most important, you will feel amazing. Most of my patients were stunned by how much more they could accomplish each day simply because they felt so much better.

Make the Cosmolecular Connection

My plan is based on what I call the *cosmolecular connection*. What do I mean by that? Perhaps you have heard of the term *cosmeceutical*, which combines the words *cosmetic* and *pharmaceutical*. First coined in the 1990s, this word applies to eye creams, anti-wrinkle agents, and other topical cosmetic products that contain biologically active ingredients that work the way medicines or pharmaceuticals do. I coined and trademarked the term *cosmolecular* to refer to nutrition, lifestyle, and skin care habits that promote beauty (and are therefore cosmetic) by producing real changes on the molecular level in the cells that form the human body.

We tend to think of our bodies as having a series of isolated compartments. The skin is one such compartment, the heart another, the liver another, and so on. I'd like to introduce you to a different understanding of the human body. Rather than thinking of it as a series of organs that function separately, I'd like you to think of it as a series of cells that function together. Human beings are a collection of cells—trillions of cells, to be precise. The smallest biological entities in the body that are capable of handling energy, cells group together to form organs—the eyes, the heart, the brain, and the skin, among others.

Every cell in your body is affected by every other cell in your body. For this reason, the largest organ in the human body, the skin, mirrors the health of the molecules, enzymes, proteins, and cells that form the body. Quite often we dermatologists are the first to notice the initial signs of internal physical ailments. People with liver disease look yellow, for example. By looking at the tongue, we can tell whether a patient has anemia. When someone has lupus, we recognize it by the butterfly rash on the skin. Studies have also linked poor digestion and low immunity to many types of skin rashes, including atopic dermatitis (often called eczema).

I'm willing to bet that this explanation probably makes perfect sense to you. I don't need to cite study after study for you to believe that your skin mirrors your internal health. You already know this from looking in the mirror. You probably have noticed that your skin doesn't look its best when you have a cold or flu. You may even have observed that your skin looks dull when you are constipated, have a headache or heartburn, or are exhausted after a stressful day. Your skin probably looks its best at a specific point in your menstrual cycle and its worst at yet another point in the cycle. If you pay close attention, you'll probably notice that your skin looks fantastic at a certain time of day and not so wonderful at another point *in the same day*. You'll even see that your skin appears more radiant when you feel joyful and more dull when you are angry, stressed, or sad. These are all examples of the skin reflecting changes going in inside the body.

STOP AGING FACT

The study of cell communication is one of the hottest areas of research. Thanks to the recent invention of highly specialized microscopes, scientists are now able to see live cells in action.

How Cells Age

As I've stated, each organ of the human body consists of groups of different types of cells, and these cells use chemical signals to "talk" to each other. These cellular communications are part of an immense and sophisticated communications network that no human-made telecommunications network can rival. Interestingly, telecommunications experts are closely studying cell communication in efforts to improve service provided by wireless phone networks.

In a healthy cellular environment, signals easily cross cell membranes, getting to their source. In an unhealthy environment, signals either don't reach their source or become distorted. Think of it as static on a phone line or dropped calls on your cell phone. Important messages do not reach their destination, preventing important bodily reactions from taking place.

Just as you have trillions of cells in your body, you have even more enzymes that trigger reactions in these cells. Enzymes are important, as your cells use them to create energy. If cellular enzymes don't function well—because your diet or lifestyle does not provide them with the optimal resources to thrive—then cells throughout your body manufacture less ATP, the energy storage molecule in all living cells. As a cell produces less ATP, it ages prematurely, causing cell mutations and increasing the formation of free radicals. This process happens everywhere in your body, including in the cells of your skin.

Enzymes all thrive within a very specific environment. If the fluids that form your body become too dry or too acidic, enzymes don't trigger the right reactions inside your cells—in the skin and throughout your body—leading to loss of elasticity, premature wrinkling, dullness, and sagging.

How Your Skin Ages

Any cosmetic dermatologist can help you get rid of wrinkles, but it takes the right diet and lifestyle to recapture the softness, smoothness, and resiliency of the skin of your youth. The Stop Aging, Start Living Plan addresses these subtle aging concerns, the ones that no dermatologist or surgeon can fix for you. The Stop Aging, Start Living Plan stops skin aging at its source—on the cellular level.

To understand what accelerates skin aging—and what stops it—you need a basic understanding of skin physiology. Your skin is made of several layers, all of which affect how quickly or how slowly you age.

Top layer. Called the *epidermis,* this multilayered section of the skin is constantly being worn down and replaced. New skin cells are "born" at the bottom of the epidermis, slowly moving upward as they age. After about twenty-eight days, these cells reach the skin's surface, die, and—if everything goes right—flake off, a process called *exfoliation.* Your skin's ability to exfoliate becomes less efficient as you age. If dead cells thicken on the skin's surface, less light can penetrate your skin, causing it to appear dull and lifeless. Sebum—a protective oil produced by the skin—also declines with age. You need sebum to seal in moisture. The less sebum you have, the drier your skin. The drier your skin, the duller its appearance.

Middle layer. The *dermis* contains blood vessels, nerves, hair

---

ASK DR. GRAF

Q: Is it true that men age more slowly than women?

A: Yes, and here's why. Compared to women, men have thicker skin and more collagen, and they produce more protective sebum. At menopause women's skin becomes even thinner, as a drop in the hormones estrogen and progesterone cause collagen synthesis and repair to drop. For these reasons, a man at age sixty will generally appear five to ten years younger than a female counterpart of the same age.

Dora Sayer Stopped Aging and Started Living!

"Dr. Graf has been my dermatologist for seven years. When I first came to her, I had been under the care of numerous other dermatologists. No matter how many treatments I got from other dermatologists, however, I never looked fresh. That was the component that was missing. The fillers worked in terms of diminishing the wrinkles and lines, but I continued to look tired and drawn. I was looking for a glow, and they weren't giving it to me. Dr. Graf changed all that.

"With Dr. Graf, it's not just about coming in and getting injected. She talks about diet, exercise, pH levels, ways to have fun, the importance of hydration, and all of the other variables that go into the creation of beautiful skin. She has changed more than my skin. She has changed my life.

"When I first started seeing Dr. Graf, I drank a lot of carbonated drinks and sodas. I controlled my weight by eating mostly protein and hardly any carbs. I was not in good shape physically. Now I'm cycling, taking Pilates classes, consuming Alkalinizing Cocktails, drinking more water, and eating more vegetables.

"Soon after my first visit, I started to see a real difference—and so could my friends and family. Over the years my skin has continued to evolve. I see changes all the time. My skin has a glow. My eyes are significantly brighter. I even smell better. My entire being has undergone a metamorphosis.

"I'm now age forty-eight. When people try to guess my age, they tell me they think I'm thirty-two. I attribute that to Dr. Graf and her skin care program."

—DORA SAYER,
  forty-eight, occupational therapist and mother of two

roots, and sweat glands. This is a thicker layer of skin and made mostly of a protein called *collagen*. This protein is important in maintaining the resilience and elasticity of skin, but with age its production declines. The less collagen in your skin, the more your skin sags and wrinkles. Another protein called *elastin* holds the collagen together, and *hyaluronic acid* surrounds collagen and elastin fibers, binding everything together and keeping the skin moist and plump. With age, levels of this acid diminish, making the skin less pliable, drier, and gaunt-looking.

Deepest layer. This layer consists mostly of fat, larger blood vessels, and nerves. It lies above the muscles and bones that anchor the skin to the body. Skin fat tends to diminish with age and facial muscles tend to atrophy, contributing to sagging. Blood vessels everywhere in the body tend to stiffen and narrow with age. When this happens to the blood vessels in the skin, the skin becomes pale and dull.

The rate of skin aging depends on many factors.

Genetics. Mom and Dad blessed you with a unique set of genes that program your cells to divide and die according to a preset clock. Many people blame their genetics for how they look and feel at a certain age. "Well, my mother had a lot of wrinkles at age forty, so that's how I'm going to look as well," they say. It's true your genetics are important. Yet much more important is how you treat your skin and your body—in other words, what you eat and what you do.

Sun exposure. The ultraviolet radiation from the sun damages the DNA in skin cells, damages collagen, and contributes to the formation of skin cancer, wrinkles, and overall skin aging. Age spots are actually a natural defense mechanism. They are no more than an accumulation of the ultraviolet-radiation-blocking pigment melanin. The skincare prescriptions in this book will help you to undo some of the damage you've inflicted on your skin over the years, lightening age spots and reducing the appearance of wrinkles.

Diet and lifestyle habits. Smoking, a poor diet, lack of exercise, stress, and many other factors can also accelerate skin aging. This book's plan will put an end to all of these age-accelerating habits. You can't change the past, but you can change the present and the future. You can stop aging now, as soon as today.

Amazing Results

Before you move on to the next chapter, I invite you to do an experiment. Take a walk downtown or at a mall or some other place populated by a lot of people and look closely at the faces around you. Who has skin that you wish you had? Who has skin that you never in a million years want?

I'm willing to bet that the answers will surprise you. You'll probably find that the two factors that most people link with aging— wrinkles and gray hair—probably don't really bother you. You'll probably spot a few sixty-plus women and men who have wrinkles and gray or white hair, but look absolutely amazing. You'll probably also see a few much, much younger people who still have few wrinkles and rich hair color but look terrible. The difference lies in skin suppleness and radiance. People who look amazing have skin that reflects light. People who look dull have skin that does not.

In this book I will suggest a very effective skin care routine that will help you not only prevent the formation of wrinkles but also create the vibrancy, radiance, and suppleness that really makes skin look amazing. After two weeks on this plan, your skin will reflect light. It will glow.

Most exciting? The longer you stay on the program, the better you will look. Each day you will wake up to look in the mirror and think that you look better than the day before. Not only will you look younger than your years, but you will smile more, laugh more, and feel as if life gets better and better every single day.

2
the pH connection

I've spent a great deal of my adult life in search of a magical elixir that would help me feel better. I searched for it for many, many years, looking in all of the wrong places. During medical school and residency—when my studies and training repeatedly required me to spend more than twenty-four hours at a time on my feet—I turned to caffeine. Whether it came in the form of coffee, caffeinated soda, or a caffeine pill, I used it. When caffeine failed me, I turned to sugar. It was always in abundant supply in the form of doughnuts at the nursing stations.

I somehow managed to physically survive medical school and my subsequent residency. After I began my private practice, my sleep habits improved, but I still felt awful. This was especially true after I started a family and found myself up in the middle of the night to soothe my son or daughter back to sleep. As a dermatologist, I knew how to disguise how I felt. With a specific skin care program and lots of well-applied makeup, I managed to look pretty good on the outside. No one ever looked at me and remarked, "Wow, you look tired." Yet at times I felt as if I'd been run over by a Mack truck, and I desperately wanted to feel better.

So I renewed my search for the magical elixir. At the time, antioxidant supplements were in style, so I ordered many different types.

Unfortunately, the supplements didn't help. They just gave me a stomachache.

I *knew* that the elixir was out there, however. I also was aware that pills were not the answer. I place a great deal of faith in the human body's ability to repair itself. I was convinced that the answer lay in something much more basic.

So I read. I read scientific studies. I studied nutrition. I looked at popular health books. I scoured the Internet. If a product claimed to reduce fatigue, I checked it out. I turned myself into a human guinea pig.

The aha moment hit me after I enrolled myself in a seven-day juice fast at the Omega Institute in Rhinebeck, New York. (Did I tell you that I tried *everything*?) I expected that the fast would be hard. I fortified my motivation by telling myself how much better I would feel once it was over and I could eat normally again. On the sixth day of the fast, however, something unexpected happened. I felt fantastic—so fantastic that I didn't think I would ever find a way to feel this good again. When I looked in the mirror I noticed something else: I *looked* fantastic. My skin was smooth. My eyes were clear. My face glowed. My cellulite was gone.

It got me thinking. I wanted to continue to look and feel this way for a long, long time, but I also knew I couldn't live on fruit and vegetable juices forever. "There must be an easier way," I thought. When I returned home, I began to dig deeply into the research about the benefits of fruits and vegetables. My research led me to pH theory. What I learned transformed my private practice. It will also transform the way you care for your skin.

First, let me put to rest any anxiety I may have created by mentioning my seven-day juice fast. *You do not have to do a juice fast or challenging detoxification program to stop aging!* Over the years, I've discovered lifestyle changes that are much easier to implement yet still provide the same transformative results. Although I highly recommend juicing (you'll find some of my favorite juicing "recipes" in chapter 10), this plan allows you to chew and crunch on real, cooked food. No fasting or 100 percent raw meals required!

Now that I've dispelled that fear, let's talk more about the importance of pH for beautiful skin. I'm actually glad that I didn't know

---

Jani Campelli Stopped Aging!

"I have youthful-looking skin and have always looked younger than my age. My problem: my skin tends to look dry. It's also sensitive, so I have scars that stem from my tomboy childhood. When I mentioned this to Dr. Graf, she told me that she could help my skin to develop a more radiant glow.

"I began using her products, taking the Alkalinizing Cocktail, and taking the mineral supplement. The fiber in the cocktail was key for me, because I've always suffered from constipation. Now I'm regular.

"When I started the program, my pH was 6; just three weeks later it was 7, and it seemed like everyone was noticing the difference in my skin. One of my girlfriends kept telling me, 'Your skin looks so brilliant. It's so moist. Usually your skin looks so dry, but now it has this glow.' It's true. My skin is milky, silky-looking. It shines. Random people now walk up to me and tell me that my skin looks beautiful. It's ridiculous.

"My scars have lightened up, too. Now I can walk around without any makeup on and my skin just shimmers."

— JANI CAMPELLI,
thirty-nine, personal trainer

---

about the importance of pH during my dark days of medical school. I'm sure my acid-producing lifestyle habits —no sleep, lots of caffeine, and poor eating habits—created a body pH that was incompatible with life! I'm convinced that I survived those years only because I had two important variables in my favor: I was young and my parents blessed me with decent genetics.

Why pH Matters

Of the many factors that influence your skin—particularly the brightness of it—pH is most important. Unbalanced pH makes your skin look dull. It also accelerates aging in cells throughout your body. In the skin, this accelerated aging reduces the amount and effectiveness of collagen (creating wrinkles and reducing elasticity), shrinks the size of facial muscles (resulting in sagging and gauntness), weakens facial bones (producing more sagging), and reduces the number and effectiveness of various types of skin enzymes (causing wrinkles, sagging, dryness, dullness, and tightness).

To understand how pH affects the skin in these ways, we need to get acquainted with some basic chemistry. If you're not a left-brained science geek like me, don't worry too much about the science. It's not my intention to put you to sleep or give you a brain cramp. You don't need to memorize the periodic table or take a course in organic chemistry to understand pH, but you do need to understand some basic jargon.

When I talk about pH, I'm talking about acidity and alkalinity, and about hydrogen. The pH of a solution is a reflection of the concentration of positively charged hydrogen ions.

Ions are simply molecules that have either a positive or a negative charge. Hydrogen ions carry a positive charge.

Acids produce hydrogen, so a low pH means a solution contains a lot of hydrogen. A solution is considered acidic if it has a pH below 7.

Bases neutralize hydrogen, so a high pH means that a solution contains less hydrogen. A solution is considered base or *alkaline* if the pH of that solution is above 7.

Okay, now you know the basic vocabulary. All liquids have a pH, and anything that contains fluid is a liquid. You may think of the human body as a solid because we all look solid on the outside, but roughly 70 percent of the human body is made of water. Fluid surrounds cells and fills up the insides of cells. Every part of your body—your organs, tissues, blood, heart, and skin—contains fluids, and these fluids all have a specific pH.

The most important thing to understand about pH is this fact: **For optimal health and functioning, most of the cells, fluids, and tissues in your body need a slightly alkaline pH.**

Cells in the outermost layer of skin (called the *epidermis*) are an exception. (Cells in the stomach are also an exception). These skin cells function best at a slightly acidic pH of 5.4. Decomposing dead skin cells create this slightly acidic pH, which helps to kill bacteria, yeast, and other organisms.

Cells in the inner layer of skin (called the *dermis*), on the other hand, function best with an alkaline pH of 7.35. This skin layer is responsible for skin strength and resilience. If pH falls too low, the cells in this skin layer stop dividing, produce fewer enzymes, stop making energy, and create less collagen. This leads directly to sagging, a dull color, and wrinkles.

ASK DR. GRAF

Q: Why do cells thrive in slightly alkaline fluids?

A: No one knows for sure, but it may have something to do with evolution. Life began in the oceans, which are full of alkaline minerals such as calcium carbonate. As one-celled life forms evolved into multicellular life forms, they did so surrounded by alkaline fluid.

Why Haven't You Heard of pH Until Now?

Many studies, dating as far back as the early 1900s, have documented the negative health effects of unbalanced pH. Yet it took many small discoveries over many years for pH theory to begin to take hold. Each small step in the right direction took years of research and technological development.

It wasn't until scientists were able to piece together a century's worth of research on cellular function that we had a clear picture of the importance of acidity on cell health, particularly on cancer cells. It has taken many more years still to show the affects of acidity on other aspects of health.

A little more than five years ago, Robert Young, Ph.D., Susan Brown, Ph.D., and a few other scientists, researchers, and physicians began suggesting that pH imbalance was the main cause of aging and poor health. These scientists theorized that low-grade acidosis caused chronic fatigue, osteoporosis (thinning of the bones), cancer, bladder infections, vaginal yeast infections, and many other diseases and conditions.

The revolutionary aspect of pH theory wasn't that acidosis was bad for health. That's a well-established fact. The day we are born, we are alkaline, but on the day we die we are filled with acidity. The revolutionary part was the idea that *acidosis caused aging,* rather than aging causing acidosis. An increasing number of physicians such as myself believe that excess acidity—from an overly acid-producing diet and/or lifestyle—accelerates aging by preventing cells throughout the body from effectively protecting themselves against metabolic damage.

Normal everyday metabolic processes form substances called free radicals. Similar to sparks flying off a fire, free radicals damage cells. All cells produce protective substances called antioxidant enzymes that can neutralize free radicals before they cause damage. Overly acidic fluids, however, allow more free radicals to form and hinder the effectiveness of antioxidant enzymes, leading to disease. Once the body becomes diseased, the problem is magnified, because acids build up even more quickly.

The importance of pH is rapidly gaining acceptance in the medical community, particularly in the area of bone health. I guarantee that this will not be the last time you hear about pH. In years to come, I predict that your family doctor will routinely test your pH, in the same way your doctor tests other health indicators such as cholesterol and glucose levels.

STOP AGING TIP

The outermost layer of skin is slightly acidic—for good reason. The acid kills organisms that cause rashes and other skin disorders.

Acidity and Aging

Acid is not universally bad. As I mentioned, some parts of the body need acidic fluids to do their jobs effectively. It's an imbalance of pH that accelerates aging. Unbalanced pH accelerates aging throughout the body, starting on the molecular level with the smallest components—enzymes, proteins, and cells. As unbalanced pH disrupts more and more cells, entire organs—including the largest organ of the body, the skin—become affected. Let's take a closer look at this sequence of events.

How pH Affects Enzymes

Each of your cells houses thousands of different enzymes, and each of these enzymes has a specific and important job. For example, the intestinal enzyme *lactase* breaks down lactose, the sugar found in dairy products. People who are lactose-intolerant do not have enough of this enzyme in their intestines and consequently cannot digest dairy products. Enzymes are important, as they control or trigger nearly all chemical reactions in the body. Unbalanced pH, however, greatly affects the health and function of enzymes. Most enzymes function optimally within a very narrow pH range of 7.35 to 7.45. When pH is too low, many enzymes do not do their jobs.

How pH Affects Cells

Low pH affects a particularly important enzyme that triggers the reaction that turns glucose (sugar) and oxygen into adenosine triphosphate (ATP), the currency that the body recognizes as energy. When oxygen reaches the cell, it must be converted into ATP before cells can use it for energy. It is similar to going to another country and having to convert your U.S. dollars to the currency of that country. With too much acid, however, cells lose their ability to make ATP because energy enzymes do not function properly. As ATP production falls off, cells age more quickly.

Acidic fluids also block ions (such as sodium, potassium, and calcium) from crossing cell membranes. When this happens, cell membranes lose their electrical charges and their ability to send and receive messages to and from other cells throughout your body and in your brain. Think of your cells as wireless phones and acidic pH as an electrical storm. As cells communicate with one another, the storm blocks and distorts their signals, resulting in static, misdials, and dropped calls. There was once a very humorous wireless phone commercial on television where static prevented callers from getting their messages across. The person on the other end of the line would hear something to the effect of "Come in a dress" instead of "He's such a pest." Inside the body, the ramifications of miscommunication are not quite so humorous. When cell communications break down, cells that should die continue to divide, causing cancerous tumors.

As if poor energy production and poor cell communications weren't enough, there's still more. Unbalanced pH also causes fluid to accumulate inside the cell. The cell's protective enzymes are also not able to function and harmful free radicals are created.

A S K   D R .   G R A F

Q: I've heard a lot about the importance of antioxidants. Are you saying that they are not important?

A: No, I'm not saying that at all. Antioxidants are vitally important, especially when pH is too low. Antioxidants neutralize harmful free radicals before they can damage cells. The problem is that it takes one antioxidant molecule to neutralize one free radical. Through the normal process of metabolism, many more free radicals are formed than you could ever neutralize with antioxidant supplements.

For this reason, you can't stop aging by taking every antioxidant supplement sold at the health food store. While they are helpful, they will never fully protect you. If your pH is too low, you can consume hundreds of antioxidant supplements and not be able to keep a lid on the extensive destruction caused by free radicals inside your body.

Your cells house natural antioxidant enzymes that are much more effective at neutralizing free radicals. For optimal health, you must create a favorable environment inside the body for cells to produce their own antioxidant enzymes—an environment with an alkaline pH.

How pH Affects Your Organs

Cells form your organs. As cells become sick and damaged, so do your organs. Almost all diseases are caused by the premature death of healthy cells. For example, the premature death of certain types of brain cells causes Parkinson's disease. The premature death of beta cells in the pancreas causes diabetes.

In addition to premature cell death, specific organs of the body are affected by unbalanced pH in a more circuitous way. Your body will expend great effort to balance blood pH. To maintain a constant blood pH of roughly 7.39, your body will draw nutrients away from the bones, skin, and organs to neutralize blood acids. In particular, the body will use alkaline salts (of the minerals calcium, sodium, potassium, and magnesium) to neutralize and eliminate acids in the blood. If you do not consume enough of these minerals to neutralize acids, your body will pull these minerals from reserves in your bones (calcium and potassium) and muscles (magnesium), weakening both. Your body will also shuttle acids out of the blood and deposit them in the fat layer just beneath the skin and in a few other areas, which leads to irritation and inflammation of these tissues.

The Fate of Our Oceans

An acidic pH affects oceans, streams, rivers, and ponds in the same way it affects the human body. You've probably heard how acid rain has killed off all forms of life in certain ponds and lakes. You may not have heard, however, how acidification is affecting our oceans. When carbon dioxide dissolves in the ocean, it creates carbonic acid (just as carbon dioxide creates carbonic acid in the fluids of the human body). Mineral salts present in sediment on the ocean floor can neutralize this acid, just as mineral salts from your bones and muscles neutralize acid in the body. The burning of fossil fuels, however, is creating so much carbon dioxide that the oceans are running short of what used to be an endless supply of mineral salts. Marine life that needs these minerals (such as corals, which use calcium to make their shells) are affected first, just as your bones are affected first when pH drops too low in the human body. As the oceans become more acidic, more marine life will perish, just as more tissues and organs in the human body perish with greater levels of acidity.

How does low pH affect your health? You'll feel tired and run-down. You'll catch one cold after another. Your muscles may ache. With increasing acidity, symptoms intensify, causing headaches, stomachaches, and excessive pain. Eventually, it results in disease. Unbalanced pH is thought to be the culprit of many degenerative and autoimmune diseases.

Here I've listed just some of the whole-body ramifications of un-balanced pH.

Germs multiply. Our bodies house thousands of tiny organisms, including bacteria, yeast, and molds. When the right kinds are in the right places in the right amounts, these organisms are not harm-ful and often are quite helpful. Beneficial bacteria in the gut help to digest our food and block toxins from entering the bloodstream.

Similar to what happens in a swimming pool or fish tank when you don't properly balance its pH, in the human body yeast multi-ply, crowding out healthy bacteria. Ramifications of yeast over-growth include vaginal yeast infections, bladder infections, skin fungus and toenail fungus, gastrointestinal upset, headaches, and fatigue.

Bladder irritation. The body will try to release excess acid through the urine. This acidic urine irritates the bladder, causing it to become inflamed. This results in painful, urgent urination. Re-search completed by the nonprofit Osteoporosis Research Project has linked unbalanced pH with an increased risk of interstitial cys-titis (also known as painful bladder syndrome). This study also showed that balancing pH with a mineral supplement provided quick relief for this often chronic condition.

Bones weaken. Before the body can excrete acids through the urine, it must raise pH with mineral salts. If it didn't, the acids would destroy the kidneys. These mineral salts generally come from bone. One recent study of nine thousand women conducted at the University of California, San Francisco found that women with chronically high levels of acid in their bodies had a greater risk for bone loss than women with normal pH levels. Another recent study determined that the foods in the typical American diet—which is extremely acid-producing in the body—may have more to do with poor bone health (osteoporosis) than lack of dietary calcium. Com-pleted at the University of Basel in Switzerland, this study split 161 women with low bone mass into two groups. One group of women took a daily potassium citrate supplement (citrate has an alkalinizing effect). Another group of women took a potassium chloride supplement, which was neutral in its effect on pH. The women who took the alkalinizing citrate supplement increased their bone mineral density by 1 percent, an effect similar to that of prescription bone-building medication. Women who took a potassium chloride supplement, on the other hand, experienced a decrease in bone mineral density by the same amount.

"In the modern diet, acid is generated from foods like dairy products, grains, and meats," wrote study author Reto Krapf, of the University of Basel. "Previous studies have found that the kidney does not quite keep up in removing this excess acid load, resulting in mildly elevated blood acidity."

Cells mutate. In the 1900s, a scientist named Otto Warburg did a series of experiments that examined the effects of acid and alkaline solutions on cell health. Studying both healthy and cancerous cells, he immersed some in an oxygen-poor, highly acidic solution, and others in a high-oxygen, highly alkaline solution. The cancer cells thrived in the low-oxygen, highly acidic environment but could not replicate well in the high-oxygen, more alkaline solution. The opposite held true for healthy cells. Warburg's research built on the knowledge of many previous studies that effectively showed how a low pH environment did one of two things: it either killed healthy cells or caused them to mutate into cancerous cells. This research later culminated in an experiment that earned Warburg the Nobel Prize in 1931.

Blood pressure rises. A study completed by researchers at Wake Forest University, the University of Texas, the University of Wisconsin, and the University of Mississippi determined that people with high blood pressure tended to have higher levels of uric acid in their blood. Uric acid is produced through the metabolism of animal protein.

How pH Affects Your Skin

You are reading this book because you care about your appearance, particularly the appearance of your skin. How does unbalanced skin pH cause you to appear older than your actual years? Let me count the ways.

Pimples and other bumps. The acid stored in the fat just underneath the skin irritates and inflames the skin. This irritation shows up as eczema and acne.

Wrinkles. Excess acidity in the skin hinders the electrical signals that skin cells use to communicate with each other as well as the cells' ability to produce ATP. These damaged cells lose their ability to produce certain types of collagen, which leads to wrinkled, sagging skin.

Gauntness. I mentioned that acidity can weaken bones. This includes the bones of the face, contributing to a gaunt, sunken appearance. Mineral loss also occurs in facial muscles, which causes these muscles to atrophy, again contributing to a gaunt appearance.

Poor skin tone and color. Unbalanced pH stiffens and narrows blood vessels, which in turn reduces blood flow to and from the skin. Less nutrition makes its way to the inner layer of the skin, creating a dull, ashen complexion. Also, your skin is loaded with enzymes that are important in triggering many types of cell reactions.

STOP AGING — NOW!

Before you turn to the next chapter, I want you to do something important. Go to the Internet, use your favorite search engine, and type in the words "pH test strips." Dozens of sites will come up. Choose a site that seems reputable (consult the appendix for my personal favorites) and order yourself some strips. If you instead choose to use the asphalt superhighway, you can also find them at most drugstores. Once your test strips arrive, begin testing your saliva pH first thing in the morning. You could get carried away with pH testing, testing your urine and even your blood. I've found that it's simplest to go by your saliva pH, along with how you feel and how you look. If your saliva pH improves (your goal is to get it between 7 and 7.5, corresponding to dark blue (on the strips) and you look and feel better, you can feel pretty certain that your lifestyle changes are working.

Among them are exfoliating enzymes, which help to ensure that dead skin cells shed naturally. When these enzymes do not work effectively, dead skin cells stay put, creating dull skin tone.

Skin cancer. Skin cells house antioxidant enzymes that defend the skin against damage by solar radiation. If acidic fluids cause these enzymes to lose their effectiveness, skin cancer cells more easily form and proliferate.

Athlete's foot. I mentioned that unbalanced pH allows certain types of germs to multiply. This results in dandruff, athlete's foot, and toenail fungus.

What Makes You Acid?

Normal cell metabolism produces a great deal of acid every day. The carbon dioxide released from cells, for example, reacts with water in the blood to form carbonic acid. Muscle cell contractions create lactic acid. Fortunately, our bodies have many natural mechanisms to buffer and eliminate these acids. The body constantly uses bicarbonate and alkaline salts to neutralize acid, and it releases weak acids when you breathe. It can release other acids through the kidneys, through urination. Finally, it can release acids through the skin, through sweating. In a healthy human being, the body stays in balance quite well. The problem is that few of us are healthy.

Most of us take care of our bodies in much the same way stereotypical fraternity brothers care for their frat houses—the fraternity house is littered with trash in the form of dirty dishes, beer bottles, soiled clothing, crumpled-up flyers, books, and papers, not to mention the near-comatose human life forms. It seems that trash enters the frat house at a rate that far exceeds the brothers' abilities to remove it. As clutter builds, the fraternity brothers don't function well. They can't find what they need when they need it. Homework goes undone. Papers go unwritten. Classes get skipped.

Your body functions much the same way. Think of acids as the beer bottles that build up in a frat house. If only the fraternity brothers were drinking beer, the house would probably stay in balance. Some pledges would get up early in the morning and pick up the bottles in a short period of time, so the house would remain relatively clean. Yet, hundreds of other people are drinking beer, too, leaving many more bottles lying around than there are housemates to remove them.

If—through an acid-producing diet and lifestyle—you create acid at a rate that exceeds your body's ability to neutralize and remove those acids through respiration, sweating, and urination, acids build up. What causes acids to build up too quickly? Too many acids build up in the body due to many factors, but most notably from the food you eat. Your body breaks down and digests food into simple absorbable components. These digested food components combine with bodily fluids to form a solution that is either acid or alkaline. Eat too many acid-producing foods (animal protein, refined sugar, coffee, cola, refined foods) and your body must work overtime to balance pH. No one knows precisely how many acid-producing foods you can eat before the fluids inside your body become too acidic, but the right breakdown is probably somewhere in the neighborhood of three to one, meaning you probably should be eating three alkalinizing foods for every one acid-producing food. Put another way, three-quarters of your dinner plate should contain alkalinizing foods, with just one-quarter containing acid-producing foods. Most people, however, do the opposite, eating three or four acid-producing foods for every one alkalinizing food. This causes problems!

STOP AGING FACT

Have you ever noticed how much more energy you have and how much better you look after vacationing at the shore? Part of this effect stems from the alkalinizing effect of ocean air. The salt in the ocean air creates alkalinizing negative ions that you inhale through your lungs. By the way, densely forested areas are equally alkalinizing.

To balance your internal pH, you must balance your diet—consuming more alkalinizing foods and fewer acid-forming foods. The Stop Aging, Start Living Plan will help you do exactly that.

In addition to your diet, a few additional factors play a role in pH balance. They include:

ASK DR. GRAF

Q: How quickly can I expect my pH to change?

A: If you provide your body with the right ingredients, your pH can change almost instantly. I test my pH frequently throughout the day. This gives me a good sense of how my diet and lifestyle habits affect my pH for the better or worse. I also have tested hundreds of patients during the past few years just before they made lifestyle changes and shortly afterward. I can tell you that pH changes quickly. Within an hour of taking a calcium-containing mineral supplement, you'll see an improvement of pH on your test strip. You'll feel the improvement earlier. Most of my patients tell me that they feel more energy instantly after taking a mineral supplement or drinking my Alkalinizing Cocktail for the first time. Within twenty-four hours, the effects of this change in pH will be noticeable. Within just two weeks, you can expect to see pH rise up to a full point.

The air you breathe. Air *should* be alkalinizing. Each inhalation *should* provide cells with alkalinizing oxygen. Each exhalation *should* rid cells of acidifying carbon dioxide. Yet if you smoke, you are inhaling carbon monoxide, which is acid-producing. If you live in a city with high amounts of air pollution, you are inhaling any number of different acid particles.

How you breathe. Your lungs release acids, but people who are anxious or under a great deal of stress tend to breathe shallowly and rapidly. They don't fully exhale, which allows stale carbon dioxide to remain in the lungs longer than it should. Indeed, relatively small changes in your breathing pattern can have a profound effect on body pH.

How you think and feel. Your body pH is also influenced by your emotions. A part of your brain called the hypothalamus is the master gland of the body, meaning that it can trigger the release of hormones from every other body gland. For this reason, your emotions can set off a chain reaction that either raises or lowers body pH. Joyous, happy, love-filled emotions tend to create alkaline-

---

ASK DR. GRAF

Q: I like to exercise. How do I know if I'm overdoing it?

A: Go by how you feel afterward. If the exercise was just right — and therefore alkalinizing — you should feel better after your exercise session than you did before your session. If, on the other hand, you overdid it, you'll probably feel worse after exercising, due to the accumulation of acids in your body.

---

forming chemical reactions in the body. Conversely, emotions filled with anger, fear, jealousy, and hate create acid-forming chemical reactions in the body. (You'll learn more about how thoughts and emotions trigger acid production in chapter 4.)

How you exercise (or don't exercise). Moderate exercise helps your body release acids by increasing your breathing rate (releasing acids through the lungs) and by making you sweat (releasing acids through the skin). If you don't exercise, you'll need to follow a more alkalinizing diet than someone who exercises regularly. Keep in mind that you can overdo it when it comes to exercise. Too much exercise can be as bad as too little. Cell metabolism in your muscles produces lactic acid. Normally, your body easily clears this acid, but if you exercise too much, this acid can build up.

The Stop Aging, Start Living Plan helps you to reduce acid buildup from all of these sources. Through an alkalinizing diet, deep breathing, and regular doses of exhilarating activity, you will balance your pH, improve your skin, and feel fantastic.

3

the digestion connection

My discovery of the importance of pH led me on the journey that culminated in this book. Once I started this fact-finding mission, I couldn't stop. The curious scientist in me wanted to know what else—in addition to pH—affected skin and cell health. My curiosity led me to the digestive tract.

I had noticed that my energy levels and skin tone and color were at their peak when my digestive system was working well. I also had noticed that I didn't look or feel my best when I felt bloated because I had wolfed down a meal without chewing it adequately.

I began asking my patients about their dietary habits. I wanted to know how much fiber they were consuming and how regularly they went to the bathroom. I also wanted to know how they were eating (standing up and rushed versus sitting down and calm) and whether they were plagued with gas, bloating, and stomach upset. As I had suspected, the patients with poor digestion did not look as good as patients with good digestion. I also noticed that patients who took steps to improve digestion—by eating more fiber, eating less antibiotic-laced meat, chewing their food more thoroughly, and eating in a more relaxed atmosphere—felt better and looked better. Aha. I was on to something. Again, I went back to science to find the connection. Sure enough, I found many reasons why digestive health affected skin health. Let's take a closer look.

Ellie Warden Stopped Aging!

I've known Dr. Graf for more than nineteen years, since I first brought my daughter to her for acne treatment. Dr. Graf gave my daughter skin that was so beautiful that I decided to see what she could do for me.

"When I made my first appointment, I was doing everything wrong. I was smoking three packs a day, eating poorly, and falling apart emotionally due to the recent death of a loved one. Dr. Graf gave me the Botox and other treatments that I requested, but she gently suggested that I should also make some lifestyle changes. One day she wasn't so subtle. She said, 'Ellie, there is not much more I can do for you cosmetically. You have to change what you are doing.'

"I listened, making small changes over time. I started with the Alkalinizing Cocktail and minerals. I actually now take the cocktail ingredients with me to work. It really keeps me going. Then I began to overhaul my diet. Rather than living off canned and prepared food that I bought at CVS and 7-Eleven, I began shopping for fresh food at the supermarket. I also changed my life, even finding a new job that better suited me. I stopped smoking, too. That was the hardest change of all, but I did it.

"Dr. Graf gave me a blueprint that I could follow to take little steps that were never overwhelming. I did all of this gradually over a four-year period, and these small, incremental changes have transformed me. Mentally and physically, I'm a new person. Now, looking back, I can see that the little steps were part of a whole plan.

"When you see the person I was and the person I now am, it's tremendous. I'm now sixty-two, but people think I'm twelve years younger. I also have more energy. I'm able to hold on to a job that is challenging both physically and mentally. I get up in the morning with so much energy. I wake up with a smile on my face."

— ELLIE WARDEN,
   sixty-two, nurse

Where Food Goes

To understand how digestion affects your skin, you first must understand what digestion is and where it starts. Digestion, simply, is what your body does to break down and use the food you eat. It starts in your mouth.

In the mouth. Your teeth and tongue mash up your food. As you chew, your salivary glands secrete enzymes that start to break down your food, beginning to transform some starches into sugar. Too often, we skip this important digestive step, gulping down huge chunks of food without chewing it first. Your stomach doesn't have teeth! As I often tell my patients, the opposite of digestion is indigestion.

In the stomach. After you swallow, your chewed food travels down your esophagus and into your stomach. Muscles along the walls of the stomach twist and turn your food, much as a washing machine twists and turns clothing during the spin cycle. The gastric juices in the stomach contain enzymes that start to break down protein into its simplest components, amino acids. The stomach empties these partially digested contents into the small intestine.

In the small intestine. Here many enzymes—secreted from the liver, pancreas, and intestinal wall—continue to break your food into its simplest components. Tiny blood vessels in your intestine absorb most of the digested food molecules—in the form of sugar, amino acids, fatty acids, cholesterol, vitamins, and minerals—bringing them into the bloodstream.

In the colon. Whatever is left travels to the colon, or large intestine, where many different microbes further break down food so the body can absorb any remaining water, minerals, and salts. These bacteria also consume some of the food remnants, producing vitamin K and some B vitamins.

Okay, so now that we've finished the physiology lesson, let's get back to the topic of this chapter—how digestion affects your skin. First and foremost, your colon is one of the main organs of elimination in the body. If it doesn't do its job, other organs of elimination—particularly the skin—must pick up the slack. For this reason alone, colon health is absolutely essential for skin health.

ASK DR. GRAF

Q: It gives me the creeps that bacteria live in my stomach and intestines. Shouldn't I just take a huge dose of antibiotics and wipe them all out?

A: That's a great question. There are more organisms living in your gut than there are cells in your body. In total, these tiny bugs collectively weigh about two pounds. If that gives you the creeps, try to think of this in another way. Many of these tiny organisms are *help ful*. They synthesize vitamins and fatty acids, neutralize toxins, and make hormones. In return, we provide them with a cozy place to live and plenty of food. In other words, they help us and we help them. Without them, you would probably suffer from chronic diarrhea, not be able to control your body pH, suffer frequent bouts of food poisoning, lose the ability to comfortably eat and digest many different types of foods, and become vitamin-deficient.

Digestion is also important for another reason. Your skin cells require many different nutrients for optimal health. For example, vitamins C and E help to protect the skin from damage caused by sun exposure, smoking, and air pollution. Vitamin A helps the skin repair itself, reducing the incidence of dry, flaky skin. The B vitamin biotin helps to form skin, hair, and nail cells. If skin cells don't receive enough of this vitamin, you can develop dermatitis (an itchy, scaly rash). Many different minerals are also important for skin health. If your digestive system does not fully break down and absorb your food, however, your skin cells may not receive all of the nutrients they need for optimal functioning.

Your digestive system, immune system, and skin are all closely linked. When you inhale pollen, dust, and spores, these particles enter the lungs. Mucus eventually washes them out of the lungs and into the stomach. Beneficial gut bacteria may signal the immune system, letting it know when to react to an allergen that you eat or swallow with your mucus. If you suffer from nasal allergies, asthma, or skin reactions, chances are good that levels of these important bacteria are too low to effectively do their job.

In one of many studies that tested this theory, researchers developed an infant formula that contained nutrients that fed healthful gut bacteria. These nutrients were similar to what is naturally found in human breast milk. Researchers gave this supplemented formula to 102 babies who were born to women with a family history of atopic dermatitis (eczema), an allergic skin rash. They gave 104 other babies formula that did not contain this supplement. During the next six months, only 10 babies who consumed the supplemented formula developed eczema, whereas 24 of the babies with the regular formula developed the condition.

Unfortunately, antibiotics destroy these good bacteria. Levels of good bacteria also naturally decline with age. When levels of good bacteria are low, levels of harmful bacteria and yeast rise. This magnifies problems, because yeast produces toxins that hinder immunity, exacerbating allergic reactions. These toxins also, by the way, affect the brain, muddling your thinking and making you moody.

Take These Bacteria and Call Me in the Morning

In addition to improved skin health, optimal levels of beneficial gut bacteria provide a number of health benefits.

Faster metabolism, lower body weight. Agriculture experts have known for years that livestock gain weight when they are given antibiotics. One of the reasons many conventional farmers routinely give antibiotics to their livestock *isn't* to prevent disease (although that's certainly one concern). It's to get the animals to gain weight more quickly. Perhaps you've even noticed this antibiotic weight gain connection yourself. Why do antibiotics cause weight gain? This isn't entirely clear, but experts at the University of Michigan believe a reduction in good gut bacteria slows the metabolism and causes the body to conserve fat.

Protection from the "stomach flu." Beneficial bacteria help to keep levels of all harmful germs in check, including the virus responsible for what we call stomach flu, with its intense vomiting and diarrhea.

Reduced risk of developing colon cancer. As beneficial gut bacteria digest certain food components, they create butyrate, a

---

STOP AGING FACT

You may find it interesting to know that researchers are hard at work looking into ways beneficial bacteria can be used to prevent various types of diseases. For example, researchers hope to one day be able to introduce certain types of beneficial bacteria into the ear canal, preventing the overgrowth of harmful bacteria that cause middle ear infections. They also hope to one day grow beneficial bacteria in the mouth, where they will keep levels of tooth-eroding bacteria in check. Someday a new field of dermatology will study probiotics of the skin and how they play a role in protecting us from our environment.

---

natural anti-carcinogen. Certain types of beneficial bacteria can also bind to and inactivate some carcinogens, inhibit tumor growth, and inhibit harmful bacteria that convert pre-carcinogens into carcinogens.

Improved cholesterol. Some research shows that optimal levels of beneficial bacteria improves triglyceride and cholesterol levels.

Better tooth and gum health. In a study completed at Malmo University in Sweden, researchers split fifty-nine participants with moderate to severe gum disease into two groups. One group took a beneficial bacteria (probiotic) supplement. The other group took a placebo (sugar pill). After two weeks, the participants who took the probiotic supplement had less plaque and less severe gum disease than participants who took the placebo.

Reduced risk of ulcers, stomach cancer, and inflammatory diseases. Despite popular belief, ulcers are not caused by stomach acid. If anything, normal levels of stomach acid may prevent ulcers by keeping levels of harmful bacteria in check. Peptic ulcers and stomach cancer are actually caused by the overpopulation of a specific type of bacterium called *Helicobacter pylori*. In 2005, Australian researchers Barry Marshall and Robin Warren won the Nobel Prize in physiology or medicine for this discovery. More recently, researchers from Uniformed Services University of the Health Sciences in Bethesda, Maryland, have shown that this harmful bacterium can escape the stomach and infiltrate the bloodstream, where it may trigger chronic inflammatory conditions such as heart disease and rheumatoid arthritis. *H. pylori* may gain a foothold in the lining of the stomach when levels of other beneficial bacteria are too low, allowing *H. pylori* to proliferate.

How to Improve Digestion

The prescriptions in *Stop Aging, Start Living* will help you to improve digestion in a number of different ways.

Eat in a calm environment. I learned the importance of this piece of advice the hard way. One day while I was eating lunch, my husband got very agitated about a family issue. As we discussed

---

STOP AGING — NOW!

Too many people have a love-hate relationship with food. We tell ourselves that we love ice cream, cookies, and other foods. Some of us may even dream about food from time to time. Yet, when we actually sit down to eat, we do everything possible to ignore what we are putting in our mouths. We read books, watch television, and converse with others at the table. We don't taste or enjoy our food.

For your next three meals, I'd like you to try an enjoyable experiment. Eat without distraction. Turn off the TV if it's usually on. Remove reading materials from the table. When you sit down, notice the food on your plate. Delight in the colorful picture and wonderful aroma. As you take each bite, chew thoroughly, turning each bite into a soft mush before swallowing. Notice how the taste and texture of your food changes as you chew it up.

You can't expect to fully notice every single bite, but try to be fully conscious of your first bite, your last bite, and the occasional bite in between. In this way you'll turn each meal into an enjoyable, sensual experience and your digestive tract will thank you later. Even if you are straying from a healthful diet, enjoy the experience rather than feeling guilty.

the matter, his temper flared. As he ranted and raved, I got more and more tense. I noticed that my food felt as if it was getting stuck in my throat. It was actually hard to swallow. Later, I had a stomachache.

On a physiological level, this makes sense. When you feel calm and relaxed, you tend to chew your food more thoroughly. Gastric and intestinal juices flow more freely when you're relaxed. Digestive muscles also more easily contract and release as they should. Also, when you feel tense or angry and consequently set off your fight or flight response, the body diverts blood away from the digestive tract and to working muscles. This slows digestion and prevents some nutrients from being absorbed.

Support beneficial bacteria. The beneficial bacteria in your gut are vitally important to the digestive process. Yet most of us continually wipe out many of these bacteria by taking antibiotics and by eating foods that support the growth of harmful gut bacteria and yeast. A diet rich in processed foods and sugar, for example, continually feeds the colonies of harmful bugs, allowing them to proliferate along the lining of your digestive tract. If you've ever baked bread or brewed beer at home, I'm willing to bet this explanation makes good sense to you—you've *seen* just how quickly yeast will multiply when given just a little bit of sugar. The yeast in the gut are no different.

ASK DR. GRAF

Q: It seems as if my digestive woes began when I started taking oral contraceptives. Could there be a connection?

A: I think you are certainly on to something. Oral contraceptives, steroids, and antacids are all known to reduce levels of beneficial bacteria in the gut.

The Stop Aging, Start Living Nutrition Prescription will help you to maximize your consumption of foods that feed beneficial bacteria, such as dark green vegetables, garlic, onions, lentils, soy, oats, and fruit. It also will help you to minimize your consumption of foods that feed yeast and other harmful organisms, including sugar and processed foods. In chapter 6, you'll also find my suggestion for an important supplement that will help you to regularly replenish levels of beneficial gut bacteria. I don't recommend many supplements, but the ones I do are vitally important to your Stop Aging efforts.

Keep food moving. Slowed digestion encourages yeast to multiply, as they love to feed on fermented food. The Stop Aging, Start Living Plan will supply you with enough fiber—both from food and from a supplement—to ensure that digested food moves through your intestines at an optimal pace.

Experiment with eating fruit first. Another strategy that may improve digestive health is food combining. William Howard Hay first introduced the theory of food combining in 1911. He and other proponents of food combining theorized that different types of food require different types of enzymes and different pH balances for proper digestion. Eat the wrong foods in the wrong combinations, the theory goes, and indigestion occurs.

From personal experience, I think some aspects of food combining make sense. It makes sense that eating fruit alone—and not in combination with other foods—would aid digestion. The body breaks down fruit more quickly than it does other foods. If you eat fruit in combination with a slow-digesting food such as meat, the fruit will sit in the stomach and intestine until the meat is digested. The longer it sits, the more it ferments, causing excess gas and bloating.

Personally, I can attest that whenever I eat fruit alone—as a between-meal snack—I feel better and have less gas than when I eat it with meals. Yet, despite the many, many years food-combining theory has been in existence, no reputable studies have been conducted that support it.

To decide whether food combining affects your digestion, I suggest you do an experiment. For two weeks, eat fruit either thirty minutes before a meal (giving your stomach and intestines time to digest and process it) or alone as a snack. Then, for two weeks, eat fruit with meals. Notice how you feel during both experiments. If you feel better when you eat fruit separately—as I and many of my patients have noticed—then it makes sense to put in the effort to keep up this lifestyle change. On the other hand, if you notice no difference, it probably doesn't make sense for you to do this. If you have diabetes or any other blood glucose disorder, stick with low-glycemic-index (slow-digesting) fruit, and check with your health care professional.

Stay hydrated. In the gut, water mixes with food, allowing it to pass through the gastrointestinal system more easily.

Stop taking antacids. Many people blame stomachaches on excess stomach acid. As a result, they take antacids day in and day out, yet their stomachaches continue to worsen and become more frequent. Is their acid really out of control? Usually it's not. It's the daily use of antacids—not the stomach acid itself—that's probably worsening their stomachaches. When scientists at the University of Michigan treated mice with drugs that blocked acid production in the stomach, the mice acquired more harmful gut bacteria and developed painful inflammatory changes in their stomach linings. Why? Because, as it turns out, stomach acid is a *good* thing (as long as it remains in the stomach and does not leak upward into the esophagus, but that is a topic for another day). Gastric acid not only helps to digest your food but also functions as a powerful antimicrobial that kills many of the bad bugs that inhabit the food you eat. When you take acid-lowering medicines, you interfere with this natural defense mechanism. Low levels of gastric acid allow bad bacteria to colonize the stomach wall, causing inflammation, which can lead to gastritis. Left untreated, gastritis can lead to ulcers and even stomach cancer.

Putting the Puzzle Together

You might think of the basic components of the Stop Aging, Start Living Plan as three jigsaw puzzle pieces. Without all of the pieces, there's a gaping hole in the puzzle. For beautiful, breathtaking skin and total body youthfulness, you must put all of the pieces together. Balancing body pH is one piece of your puzzle. Good digestion is another. Turn the page to discover the final puzzle piece, so you can begin assembling your picture of more youthful radiant skin.

4

the joy connection

A few years ago, I attended a party at a friend's house. I traveled three days by car to get to the party, and I had an awful time. As I walked around the party with a drink in my hand, I began to feel more and more annoyed. I was sour. I was angry for taking three days out of my life to attend a party that I didn't find enjoyable. The wine in my glass didn't even taste good.

As I stood there looking at the other party goers, I wondered, "When was the last time I really had fun?" I thought for a while, but I couldn't remember. I felt emotionally exhausted. As I got dressed and ready to go out on any given night, I had to force myself through the motions.

Fun and joy were missing from my life. In that moment, the aha hit me. I realized that positive emotions such as joy, love, and happiness were just as important to youthful skin as digestion and pH. I began to think about the faces of people I knew. I realized that the grumps in my life didn't look good. Besides the nearly constant frowns on their faces, they were lacking a glow. They looked like wax models of themselves. Then I thought of the most joyful people I knew. They smiled a lot, and they looked as if they had swallowed a lightbulb and it was shining light through their skin.

I thought about the huge wireless network of cells that formed the human body. I wondered, "How do emotions, feelings, thoughts, and stress affect cells in the skin?" The question led me back many years, to my early days as a physician researcher, when I worked in the labs of the National Institutes of Health.

Lisa Kaplan Stopped Aging!

"I first met Dr. Graf when I tagged along with my sister to her dermatologist appointment. I was going through a bad time in my life, and Dr. Graf could tell just by looking at me. She said, 'I can make you look happier.' She did, and I was hooked.

"That was in 1997, and I've been a regular patient of hers ever since. I use the skin care products that she recommends to me, take the Alkalinizing Cocktail, and follow just about any other advice she's given to me over the years. One time I came in with my face somewhat swollen, and she suggested I start drinking more water. That was something I knew I should be doing, but I had always been lazy about it. Because everything she had ever told me had worked, I knew I just had to do it. I've been drinking more water ever since.

"Her advice has allowed me to put off plastic surgery. My skin is clearer than it has ever been. When I first started seeing her, it alternated between being very greasy and very dry. Now it's normal. My skin looks groovier, I feel prettier, and I have a brighter look on my face. She makes me feel the best I can. I'm turning fifty, but I don't look anywhere near it, and I know it's from her program. I was out the other day with my middle daughter, who is seventeen, and someone asked me if I was her sister. My kids think I look great, and I know they love showing me off to their friends because I look young."

—LISA KAPLAN,
    fifty, full-time mom of four teenage children

You Look How You Feel

As a research scientist for the National Institutes of Health, I developed a fascination with peptides. These tiny fragments, composed of five to ten amino acids, form an intricate signaling system inside the body. The work that my lab colleagues and I performed on peptides was published in the prestigious journal *Science* and resulted in an NIH patent, but even more important, it revealed to me the awesome world of the most elaborate and brilliantly designed wireless communications network ever created. As I've mentioned before, the cells in your body "talk" to one another constantly. Peptides enable this communication to take place. Candace Pert, Ph.D., a colleague of mine at the NIH, described the nature of peptides so perfectly in her book *Molecules of Emotion* that I won't attempt to outdo her. As she put it, in the body, "amino acids are the letters. Peptides . . . are the words made from these letters. And they all come together to make up a language that composes and directs every cell, organ, and system in your body."

Neuropeptides link the health of the brain (emotions, moods, thoughts, feelings, brain waves, memories) with the health of the skin. A neuropeptide is a type of peptide that originates in the brain and nervous system. These peptides are responsible for our feelings—anger, sadness, joy, contentment, and courage. They communicate messages that enable the brain to control energy, pain, pleasure, and even body weight. They form memories, help you solve problems, and regulate immunity.

STOP AGING FACT

When you scratch yourself—even if you're not feeling particularly itchy—the scratching stimulates nerves in the skin, which in turn stimulate immune cells. These immune cells travel to the brain, where they secrete inflammation-producing substances (called cytokines). The cytokines tell the brain, "Itchy!" The brain responds by releasing specific peptides that relay signals back to the skin, creating an itchy sensation. This is why scratching what at first feels like a localized itchy spot on your arm tends to create itchy sensations over a wider area, sometimes even all over your body. I bet you are starting to feel a little itchy just reading about it!

Neuropeptides circulate long distances, traveling through spinal fluid, nerves, blood, and other bodily fluids. You might think of them as the teenage gossip spreaders, as their messages tend to be contagious. Just as one popular and charismatic teenager can quickly affect what many other teens choose to do in their free time, wear, and eat, one neuropeptide can cause many different reactions in many different cells throughout your body.

Skin cells—along with cells in the nervous system, gastrointestinal tract, and immune system—contain countless neuropeptide *receptors*. These molecules receive messages from neuropeptides, which in turn provide skin cells with important messages about how they should function. Based on these neuropeptide messages, skin cells react by sending out their own peptides to surrounding skin cells. In this way the message of joy in the brain can be relayed to the skin, which reacts by sending out peptides that cause the skin to glow. Similarly, we blush when we are embarrassed. We sweat when we're nervous. The skin looks pale when we're scared. The skin glows when we're in love. These skin changes are the brain's way of broadcasting these emotional states to the outside world.

By the way, the peptide communications network operates in both directions. What happens in the brain affects the skin, and what happens in the skin affects the brain. So, as the skin begins to glow, it sends messages back to the brain, which intensify the sensation of joy. You feel good when you look good, and you look good when you feel good.

STOP AGING FACT

Substance P, a neuropeptide released from the nerves during times of stress, stimulates the proliferation of the sebaceous glands in the skin to produce more oil, which contributes to acne.

Depending on the nature of these neuropeptide and skin peptide communications, cells in your skin will make more or less collagen and elastin, which in turn leads to either youthful, plumped-up skin or wrinkled, older-looking skin. It'll either repair scars or allow scars to thicken. Your circulatory system will either increase or decrease blood flow to your skin, creating either a breathtaking radiance or a dull pallor.

Your Skin Can Hear You Now

I don't know about you, but I personally use many different methods to communicate with others long distance. I use my cell phone, which sends wireless messages—somewhat like the way your body uses peptides. I can use my landline, which sends fiber-optic information through wires, just as the nerves of the body communicate the sensations of pain, temperature, pressure, motion, tension, and texture to the brain. Or I could send an e-mail, which is capable of broadcasting a message to many different people, in much the same way the brain and body use electricity to communicate various messages to cells.

Every part of your body is immersed in and generates vibratory information. The molecules that form the cells in your body spin, wiggle, and shake millions of times each second, and these vibrations communicate important information to the cell and to other cells. Every cell in your body is surrounded by an electrical field, created by the flow of positively charged potassium ions and negatively charged chloride ions across membranes. If these fields are disrupted, you have an acceleration of aging and disease. In the skin, in particular, these currents attract repair cells to damaged areas, orchestrating wound healing.

Bioelectrical fields function on a set rhythm that is largely in sync with the natural rhythms of the universe. These circadian rhythms cause cells to function differently during the day than they do at night. For example, cells in the skin go into protective mode during the day, secreting substances that protect the skin from sunlight and air pollution. At night, they—along with the rest of the body—go into renewal mode, repairing damage.

In addition to these day and night rhythms, the bioenergy of various parts of your body follows other longer or shorter rhythms. Brain waves, for example, tend to react to surrounding weather energy, slowing down just before an electrical storm and speeding up during sunny weather (which may explain why you can sometimes find it more difficult to focus during bad weather).

The pharmaceutical industry is hard at work trying to map out the intricate networks that link the skin and brain (not to mention the brain and immune system, brain and gastrointestinal tract, and brain and circulatory system). You see, pharmaceutical companies are well aware of the effects of optimal cell communications (optimal health and well-being) and suboptimal communications (disease). In years to come, we'll have much more knowledge about how these communications networks work, and we'll have drugs and products available that will stop the transmission of signals that age the skin and encourage the transmission of signals that beautify that skin.

STOP AGING TIP

Choose skin care products and makeup that smell as wonderful as they make you look. The nose taps into the same wireless network as the skin, relaying information about scent to the brain. Research shows that odors tend to have a strong and immediate effect on humans. It's possible that skin care products that smell good can also make you feel good, which, in turn, will help you to look good. Conversely, skincare products that smell bad make you feel bad, which makes you look bad!

Stress Accelerates Aging

Okay, so now you understand the wireless and wired networks that connect the brain to the skin. Let's take a closer look at what disrupts these networks. In a word, I'm talking about stress. When I talk about stress, I'm not just talking about emotional stress. I'm talking about anything that causes the body's *stress response* (humans' built-in way of responding to threatening situations) to override and overpower your body's *relaxation response* (humans' built-in mechanism for stress recovery). By this definition, stress includes chronic negative thoughts ("I just know I'll never be able to measure up"), negative emotions (sadness, depression, fear, loneliness, frustration, anger, anxiety, worry, and so on), negative physical sensations (extreme cold or heat, pain, or the physical exhaustion caused by lack of sleep or extreme exercise), negative sensory stimuli (extremely loud noises, extremely unpleasant smells), and negative body reactions (infection, fever).

When any of these factors trigger the stress response, your adrenal glands release adrenaline (also known as epinephrine) and other hormones, increasing your breathing, heart rate, and blood pressure. This ensures that more blood reaches the brain and muscles, so you can more easily fight or flee. Adrenaline also causes a rapid release of glucose and fatty acids into your bloodstream, so your muscle cells have plenty of energy to burn. During stress, your senses and memory will sharpen and you will be less sensitive to pain. All unnecessary bodily functions shut down. Growth, reproduction, and the immune system all go on hold. Blood flow to the skin and digestive tract is reduced.

If your stress response kicks in only when it should—during a

---

ASK DR. GRAF

Q: I never thought of loud noise as a stressor. How does noise set off the stress response?

A: Humans evolved thousands of years ago to fear loud noises. For our ancient ancestors, the loudest noises were often associated with something life-threatening — the roar of a wild animal, the clap of thunder, the scream of a child as she is being mauled by a wild animal. Today, not all loud noises are life-threatening. Other than hurting your hearing, a rock concert isn't going to do you bodily harm. Yet your body still interprets these noises as stressful and sets off the stress response. Also, chronic low-level noise (such as the noise you would hear day in and out if you lived near a busy highway) has been linked with high blood pressure, peptic ulcers, cardiovascular deaths, strokes, low immunity, and learning disabilities.

true life-threatening situation such as trying to suddenly maneuver your car around an obstacle at high speed—and your relaxation response kicks in shortly afterward, your body remains in equilibrium. The problem is that many of us tend to initiate our stress response repeatedly during times when we don't need it. We also—through the use of caffeine and other stimulants—suppress our relaxation response.

YOUR BRAIN ON CORTISOL

When you activate your stress response chronically, the stress hormone cortisol remains elevated. This hormone is particularly harmful when it remains in certain parts of the body longer than it should. In the brain, this hormone interferes with peptides and other chemical messengers. By preventing brain cells from communicating with one another, cortisol causes confusion. This is why some people's minds literally go blank during a crisis. It is also why some people find themselves at a loss for words when they are nervous or under stress.

Over time, chronically elevated cortisol levels can damage the hippocampus, the part of the brain in charge of learning and memory. This muddles your thinking, impairs your memory, and may even be a factor in age-related dementia and Alzheimer's disease.

Cortisol and other stress hormones are equally damaging to other parts of the body. For this reason, chronic stress has been linked to just about every disease you can think of, including heart disease, cancer, high blood pressure, peptic ulcers, asthma, diabetes, and osteoporosis. It also has been linked to muscle weakness, muscle tension, infertility, impotence, GI distress, headaches, and fatigue.

As it turns out, stress ages every part of your body—from head to toe and all of the skin in between—in three important ways.

By aging your cells. Researchers at the University of California, San Francisco have determined that chronic stress injures important parts of the cell called telomeres, DNA segments found at the ends of the cell's chromosomes. Over a cell's lifetime, the telomeres naturally shorten as the cell repeatedly divides. When the telomeres become too short, the cell stops dividing and eventually dies.

STOP AGING FACT

Emotional stress usually starts in your mind with a thought ("There's no way I'll get this project done on time! My partner is going to be so mad at me"). The thought produces an emotion — fear, anger, guilt, frustration, irritation, anxiety, sadness, and so on. The emotion triggers physical changes in the body — crying, shallow breathing, muscle tension, chest tightness, sweating, dry mouth, and others. These physical changes outlast the mental triggers. Long after your thoughts have returned to those of a more positive nature and long after the negative emotion has subsided, you may still feel muscle tension, have an upset stomach, or experience other physical signs of stress.

Stress accelerates telomere shortening by reducing the activity of a protective enzyme called telomerase. Stress also increases oxidative stress, which directly damages DNA. Both interactions cause telomeres to shorten more quickly, accelerating cell aging and cell death.

By lowering body pH. Many years ago, Herbert Benson, a cardiologist at Harvard Medical School, conducted a number of studies looking at the physiological differences between stressed-out study participants and relaxed study participants. He found that people under stress not only had faster heart rates, high blood pressure, and increased breathing rates than when they were relaxed, they also produced more carbon dioxide and lactic acid, both markers of increasing acid levels in the body. This makes sense physiologically, as the stress response stimulates the adrenal glands to speed up the body's metabolic activity. With this increase in cell metabolism comes an increase in metabolic by-products that create acids. Skin cells may be most affected, as the stress response redirects blood flow away from skin and to the working muscles. This hinders the skin's ability to eliminate metabolic acids. As these wastes build up, the pH of the deeper layers of skin drops.

By affecting digestion. Stress may worsen digestion by affecting levels of gut bacteria. In an experiment conducted at McMaster University in Ontario, Canada, researchers repeatedly subjected rats to different types of stress over a period of ten days. For instance, in one experiment the thirsty rats were placed on a platform surrounded by water, but they couldn't actually drink it. After the conclusion of the experiment, researchers examined the rats' gut tissue. The repeated stress increased the amount of harmful bacteria colonizing the gut wall. It also made the gut wall more permeable, so these harmful bacteria could more easily infect nearby lymph nodes.

STOP AGING FACT

How do you react to stress? Do you bite your nails? Scratch your face? Pick at a spot on your arm? Many people do. Why? When you feel anxious, your body releases histamines. In addition to worsening allergic reactions, histamines make you feel itchy.

STRESS AND YOUR SKIN

Okay, now let's take a look at what stress does to your skin. Let me warn you: it's not pretty. If you are under chronic stress, you can expect to see the following negative effects.

Itchy, ugly rashes. Your epidermal skin cells lie on top of each other and are packed tightly together, forming a strong barrier that blocks the penetration of bacteria and other pathogens. When you are under stress, however, this protective outermost layer of skin becomes impaired.

In one study, researchers examined the skin of twenty-seven students in three situations: just after returning from winter vacation (low stress), during final exams (high stress), and during spring break (low stress). Stress caused the outermost layer of skin to break up as skin cells shrank and the lipids between these cells evaporated. These tiny cracks make the skin more permeable, allowing harmful bacteria, particularly a type called *Staphylococcus aureus,* to infiltrate the deeper layers of skin. These bacteria produce a protein that activates the immune system, leading to eczema and psoriasis.

More severe acne. In one study, researchers at Stanford

University examined the severity of acne in twenty-two college students during final exam week. Students who were more highly stressed by their exams had worse acne than calmer, less stressed students. In other research, relaxation therapies such as psychotherapy and biofeedback have been shown to reduce the severity and incidence of acne.

More deadly skin cancers. In studies done on mice at Johns Hopkins University, chronic stress sped the formation of skin cancer when mice were exposed to ultraviolet light. In a different study completed at Yale University, people with melanoma, the deadliest form of skin cancer, were more likely to have gone through stressful life events such as a divorce, personal bankruptcy, or period of unemployment during the years leading up to their diagnosis than people who did not have skin cancer.

Less severe dermatitis. The stress hormone cortisol acts as a powerful steroid that shuts down one part of the immune system (making you more susceptible to colds and flu) but cranks up another part, making you more susceptible to allergens. In a Japanese study of twenty-six patients with atopic dermatitis (an allergic inflammation of the skin), patients experienced a reduction in their symptoms— even when they were exposed to the allergen that triggered them— for two hours after watching a funny movie. The laughter produced by the movie probably reduced levels of stress hormones.

Cold sores. Stress affects many different immune cells negatively, which causes flare-ups of immunity-related skin conditions such as cold sores (along with psoriasis, eczema, shingles, and viral warts).

Frown lines. Repeated frowning causes frown lines, and most people frown without knowing it. You can *try* to will yourself to smile, but if you are under chronic stress or have many negative thoughts and emotions, these forced smiles won't last. Indeed, a natural, long-lasting smile comes only from positive emotions that make you *want* to smile.

Dryness. Stress reduces the lipid barrier on the skin, allowing fluids to evaporate and leading to dryness.

Dullness. When the stress response kicks in chronically, skin cells take longer to reach the skin surface and flake off, allowing dead skin cells to build up and causing your skin to look dull.

How to Think Young

So now you understand how stress and negative emotions age your skin. What can you do about it? Do you need to check yourself into an ashram for a month of meditation and prayer? Probably not.

My joy-producing, stress-releasing prescription is much simpler, faster-acting, and a real pleasure. It involves regularly dosing yourself with rip-roaring fun. Let me explain.

During the weeks that followed my terrible party experience described at the start of this chapter, I spent a lot of time thinking about joy and fun. I kept asking myself about the last time I'd really had fun. As I mentioned, the answer eluded me for a few weeks.

Then one day it hit me. I remembered my college days as a pre-med student. At this time of my life, I looked forward to getting out of bed each morning. I smiled contagiously. I had energy. I felt good. I looked great.

What made the difference? During this time of my life, I danced. I took classes and was a member of a student dance company. I loved it.

In that moment I realized that dance was the joy that was missing.

STOP AGING — NOW!

Treat yourself to a good belly laugh. What makes you laugh? Do you have a friend who often tells uproarious stories? Do you enjoy comedy? Do you have a favorite funny movie? Laughter goes a long way toward reducing stress. Researchers at Loma Linda University have shown that endorphins (a type of neuropeptide that produces sensations of euphoria and numbs pain) and human growth hormone (which seems to optimize immunity) levels rose and stress hormones fell — for as long as twenty-four hours — after study participants watched funny movies. Even anticipating watching a funny movie — without actually watching it — caused this positive brain chemistry response.

So, in my forties, I decided to bring dance back into my life. I signed up for a dance class and began dancing each morning to songs on the radio. Now I look forward to getting up each morning. I smile contagiously. When I dance, I'm alive.

For you it might be dance or it might be something else. You might find joy in yoga and meditation. You might find joy in a more active pursuit, such as cycling or running. You might find it in sculpting or painting. You might find it in singing. What works for one person doesn't work for someone else. So don't beat up on yourself for still feeling stressed at the end of a yoga class while everyone else looks blissed out. That only means that yoga isn't for you.

For the moment, don't worry about figuring out the one thing that will bring you joy. Just let the seed germinate as you continue to read this book. Eventually, when you get to the Stop Aging Lifestyle Prescription in chapter 7, that seed will have taken root. The advice you'll find in that chapter will help you to water and care for it, so it sprouts into the perfect idea of how to infuse your life with more joy and less stress.

part 2

Now that you know how pH, digestion, emotions, and other factors affect aging, let's get to what you really want to know—what to do about it all. To stop aging and start living, you will use four key Stop Aging prescriptions:

1. The Stop Aging Nutrition Prescription, to improve pH, digestion, brain health, and cell energy and communication

2. The Stop Aging Supplement Prescription, to optimize your body on the days you can't eat as well as you should

3. The Stop Aging Skin Care Prescription, to heal, beautify, brighten, hydrate, and soften the skin on your face and body from the outside in

4. The Stop Aging Lifestyle Prescription, to improve your body's natural detoxification system and strengthen your relaxation response

When added together, these prescriptions will help you look and feel younger. Not only will your skin look more radiant and become softer and smoother, you will feel more energetic and joyful. The Stop Aging 2-Week Plan outlined in chapter 9 will walk you through the four Stop Aging prescriptions step by step. Each day, you'll find detailed examples of what to eat, along with reminders to help you put your skin care, lifestyle, and supplement prescriptions into practice.

5

the stop aging
nutrition prescription

The Nutrition Prescription gently, conveniently, and deliciously helps you transform your diet from one that creates acidity to one that allows your body to optimize pH. By encouraging you to increase your consumption of the most powerfully nutritious foods on the planet, the Nutrition Prescription will help you improve digestion, increase

---

ASK DR. GRAF

Q: I've been living on fast food, steak, coffee, and junk food for years. Am I a lost cause?

A: Listen, no one was more of a nutritional train wreck than I was! I changed my diet and improved my pH, so I know you can, too. It's never too late to do something good for your body. It doesn't matter how much junk you've eaten over the course of your life, how little you've paid attention to your skin, or how stressful your lifestyle has become. As soon as you take charge of your beauty and health, your cells respond. Your organs, tissues, and cells want to work with you. Your body craves pH balance. Give your cells the ingredients they need to function optimally and that's exactly what they will do.

your production of joy-producing neuropeptides, and improve cell energy and communication.

Eat as Your Ancestors Ate

The Nutrition Prescription will help you adopt a diet that more closely resembles the natural diets of our very ancient ancestors. More than a million years ago, our ancestors ate only foods that they could find on nearby plants, bushes, and trees. Researchers who have studied the fossilized remains of early humans have determined that these ancient humans' diets consisted primarily of leafy greens, fruit, seeds, and roots, with occasional wild game. The human body evolved on this diet, which is probably why fruits, vegetables, tubers, and seeds are among the most health-promoting foods on the planet.

Now, don't let this information scare you. This isn't a vegetarian diet. This isn't a raw food diet. You can indeed eat meat and other cherished foods on this plan. The Nutrition Prescription requires only that you stay in balance. Unfortunately, most of us are woefully out of balance. Today, most humans consume a diet that is the complete opposite of how our ancient ancestors ate. Whereas our ancient ancestors probably ate more than ten daily servings of fruits and vegetables, the Centers for Disease Control estimate that more than 75 percent of Americans eat fewer than five daily servings, and these servings often come in the form of ketchup and french fries.

What are we eating instead? Lots of animal protein, lots of refined wheat products, and lots of added sugar in the form of sodas, snack foods, and sweet treats. Vegetables, once our main course, are now our garnishes.

This dietary mismatch between what we eat and what our bodies actually need lowers pH, hinders digestion, and blocks cell signaling throughout the body and in the brain. As a result, we're accelerating the aging process not only in the skin but throughout the body. Study after study consistently shows that the American diet, with its lack of fruit and vegetables and heavy emphasis on sugar and meat, contributes to memory loss, cancer, heart disease, obesity, and much more.

Eating for pH Balance

In this chapter, you will find my list of top alkalinizing Age Stoppers along with my list of acid-producing Age Accelerators. The Age Stoppers are true power foods. Not only are these foods highly alkalinizing, they also improve digestion, cell communication, and brain function. The Age Accelerators, on the other hand, do the opposite. They lower pH, hinder digestion, make you moody, and muddy concentration. Before we get to the Age Stoppers and Age Accelerators, however, I need to explain a little science about how the food you eat affects your pH.

Most of us think of foods as acid or alkaline based on their pH outside the body. In other words, we tend to think of acidity based on how a food tastes. *Sour* and *bitter* foods tend to be acidic outside the body. The more sour a food tastes, generally the lower its pH. Lemon juice, which is very sour, is a 2.1 on the pH scale outside the body. Orange juice, which is less sour, is a 3. Coffee, much less sour, is a 5.

Here is where things get confusing for most people. Some foods that are *acidic-tasting* (lemons, for example) are actually *alkalinizing* inside the body. Some foods that are alkaline outside the body are acid-producing inside the body. Here's what's going on. When you eat, your stomach and intestines break food down into its simplest components. Every food contains many different components, some of which are alkalinizing and some of which are acidifying. For example, 1 cup of wild rice contains 7 grams of protein, which is acid-producing in the body. It also, however, contains 3 grams of fiber, some iron, and trace amounts of additional alkalinizing minerals. If a food—such as wild rice—contains more alkalinizing components than acidifying ones, it raises body pH. It's considered an alkalinizing food. If it contains more acidifying components than alkalinizing ones, it lowers pH. It's considered an acid-producing food.

Some of the early promoters of pH balance recommended diets that were almost completely devoid of acid-producing foods. These diets consisted of raw vegetables, seeds, avocados, specific low-sugar fruits, and nuts. They included no meat, no coffee, no processed foods, and very little in the way of cooked foods, grains, or sugar-containing fruit. Although such diets are undoubtedly nutritious, I don't know anyone who has had the courage to sustain such a huge dietary change.

The good news is that an extreme diet like this is unnecessary to balance pH. In my experience in working with hundreds of patients, you can raise body pH with a much more reasonable and delicious diet that includes roughly three alkalinizing foods for every one acid-producing food. You may even be able to get by with a two-to-one ratio, and once you get in pH balance you may be able to maintain pH with a one-to-one ratio. Finding what works for you may take some trial and error, and if you're so inclined, you can test your pH each morning and after meals to see how foods affect your pH. Once you have your test strips, this process is very easy and fast. You just tear off a strip, wet it with your tongue for a second, and compare the color on the strip to a color chart to read your pH.

If you'd rather not test your pH every morning, however, then err on the side of caution and aim for a three-to-one ratio. The Stop Aging menus in chapter 9 and recipes in chapter 10 are based on this ratio, so you can lean on this information to see what three-to-one eating looks like.

Stay Young with Organic Foods

When you eat conventionally grown foods, you accelerate aging due to the following factors.

You ingest harmful pesticide and herbicide residue. More than four hundred chemicals are regularly used in conventional farming to kill weeds, insects, and other pests that attack crops. Although farmers and food processors regularly wash produce after picking, research shows that some of these chemicals linger. Researchers who have tested various types of grocery store produce have determined that between 1 and 17 percent of the original pesticide residue remains on any given fruit or vegetable even after the processor has thoroughly washed it. The ingestion of these residues has been linked with a range of conditions, including cancer, reduced fertility, chronic fatigue syndrome in children, and Parkinson's disease.

You end up with fewer plant nutrients. Organic foods generally contain more beneficial plant nutrients than conventionally grown foods. The more stress a plant undergoes (drought, pests, excessive sunlight), the more phytochemicals the plant must produce to ward off pests, and these phytochemicals are natural antioxidants that improve our health when we eat them. Danish researchers have found that organic crops contain 10 to 50 percent more antioxidants than conventional crops.

You're eating tainted meat. When you eat the meat of conventionally grown animals, you may be ingesting small amounts of antibiotics and hormones, which may negatively affect your health in many different ways (including reducing levels of beneficial gut bacteria).

I realize that it may not be realistic to consume only organic foods. Your grocery store may not stock organic options for every food you consume, or you may find that you can't afford to go 100 percent organic. Do the best you can, using the following tips for guidance when purchasing conventionally grown foods.

• Buy conventionally produce only when it's in season, and if possible purchase it from a local farmer. Farmers can usually get by with fewer pesticides and other chemicals if they do not need to ship foods across the country.

• Remove the tops of celery and outer leaves of lettuce, which tend to contain the most pesticide residue.

• Before eating, immerse produce in cold, clean drinking water. Scrub it if possible, but do not use soap, as soap leaves its own harmful residue.

• Trim the fat from meat, and fat and skin from poultry and fish. Animals consume some pesticides in their feed. These chemicals can make their way into the meat of the animal, but they usually become concentrated in fat just under the skin's surface rather than in the lean muscle tissue.

Finally, the following foods tend to contain the highest amounts of pesticide residue and are best eaten organic: strawberries, bell peppers, spinach, apples, cherries, peaches, cantaloupe, celery, apricots, green beans, grapes, raisins, grape juice, cucumbers, pears, winter squash, and potatoes.

Alkalinizing Age Stoppers

In the following pages, you'll find eleven foods, beverages, and spices that will help you to stop premature cellular aging. These foods will improve digestion and health, improve neuropeptide communications, improve cell energy and signaling, and decrease your risk of age-related diseases.

DARK LEAFY VEGETABLES

STOP AGING PRESCRIPTION: 1 CUP OF DARK LEAFY GREENS A DAY
Greens such as kale, collards, dark lettuces (for example, romaine and mesclun mix), endive, mustard greens, turnip greens, and dandelion greens are among the most alkalinizing foods on the planet. They also provide a rich source of vitamins such as beta-carotene, which the body converts to vitamin A. Not only does beta-carotene protect against cancer, heart disease, and cataracts, but it also is vitally important to skin health.

Greens are also a rich source of minerals. A cup of greens contains almost as much calcium as a cup of milk and as much iron as a small steak.

Greens contain plenty of plant nutrients (called phytonutrients) that ensure good health. The phytonutrients lutein and zeaxanthin in greens are the plant's natural sunscreen. These nutrients protect plant leaves from ultraviolet radiation damage. When you eat the greens, the phytonutrients in the leaves make their way into your bloodstream and into cells throughout your body. In skin cells, they protect against skin cancer. In the eyes, they protect against cataracts.

In addition to these nutrients, greens also, of course, contain chlorophyll. Chlorophyll is the chemical in plants that initiates photosynthesis (the process of turning sunlight, water, and carbon dioxide into sugar). Photosynthesis involves countless chemical reactions that can damage plant cells. Chlorophyll acts as a protective buffer, protecting plant cells from damage. It also protects plant leaves from the potentially damaging effects of sunlight, which is why the leaves most exposed to the sun tend to be the greenest. When you eat leaves that are rich in chlorophyll, the chlorophyll protects *your* cells from damage, too.

STOP AGING FACT

The more light a plant is exposed to, the more chlorophyll it needs. For this reason, the darker, outer leaves of lettuce are more healthful than the paler inner leaves.

If you have questions about how to prepare and cook greens, I have answers. Greg Thompson, a good friend of mine who happens to be the executive chef at Morton's The Steakhouse in South Park, Charlotte, North Carolina, and manager of many other Morton's kitchens, designed most of the recipes you'll find in chapter 10. Greg certainly knows his way around the kitchen. He's the person who trains *other* chefs of the various new Morton's restaurants that open around the world. He's also personally made dinner for many

---

ASK DR. GRAF

Q: I noticed you did not list spinach with the other greens. Why not?
A: Unlike other greens, spinach and chard contain weak acids that your body may or may not be able to metabolize. On the plus side, these greens also provide powerful health-promoting antioxidants. Although these weak acids are not nearly as destructive as those generated by sugar and other Age Accelerators, I decided not to list spinach along with other greens in order to encourage you to expand your greens palate. When cooking at home, experiment with unfamiliar greens such as kale and bok choy. Think of spinach as a treat for when you eat out. It's often one of the only greens available on restaurant menus.

---

famous people, such as former President George H. W. Bush and his wife, Barbara.

He and nutrition expert Leslie Dantchik, who also helped with the recipes and menus, know greens inside and out. Their recipes and menu suggestions helped me to include more greens in my daily diet, and if they could do this for *me,* I know their recipes will help *you.* You'll learn how to quickly and tastily cook any type of greens as a side dish. More important, you'll find many delicious ways to sneak more greens into all of your favorite foods.

OTHER ORGANIC VEGETABLES

STOP AGING PRESCRIPTION: 2 CUPS A DAY

Most vegetables (exceptions include corn, peas, rhubarb, string beans, and conventionally grown carrots) alkalinize the body. They also contain many different phytochemicals that have been shown to reduce risk for many different diseases, including heart disease, cancer, GI diseases, stroke, high blood pressure, asthma, and diabetes.

Why are vegetables so protective? Like dark leafy greens, vegetables contain powerful antioxidants. Vegetables also contain decent amounts of fermentable fiber. Our digestive enzymes can't break down this type of fiber, so this part of the plant passes intact into the colon, where intestinal bacteria break it down. Considered a natural "pre-biotic," plant fiber feeds beneficial bacteria in the colon.

As I mentioned earlier, vegetables—particularly when eaten raw—contain plant enzymes that help your body more fully digest food. Heat destroys these enzymes, which is why it's important to eat some of your foods raw. You don't, however, want to eat *all* of your vegetables raw, as cooking helps your body to more easily ab-

---

STOP AGING TIP

When adding more vegetables to your plate, don't forget root vegetables such as yams, sweet potatoes, jicama, rutabaga, turnips, parsnips, and kohlrabi. These root vegetables are all highly alkalinizing and rich in health-promoting phytochemicals.

sorb specific antioxidant compounds. For example, researchers from many different institutions in Europe have found that the gut absorbs five times more carotenoids from cooked carrots than from raw carrots. The absorption rate, by the way, goes up when the carrots are mashed, which provides yet another reason to chew your food thoroughly.

I'm not a natural fruit or vegetable eater. I put in a busy day at the office, so it's hard to eat as many fruits and vegetables as I know I should. The following advice has helped me to increase my consumption of fruits and vegetables. I hope it helps you, too.

• Snack on produce. If you are looking for some crunch, try sliced carrots, radishes, cucumber, broccoli, or celery. If you need something sweet, try a kiwi or a bowl of berries.

• Eat a salad with lunch and dinner. Bagged, prewashed organic salad mixes make salad creation simple and easy.

• Stock your refrigerator and freezer with microwavable veggies. Many types of veggies now come in microwavable bags. You simply take them from your fridge or freezer, puncture the bag with a fork, insert it into the microwave, and cook for five minutes.

• Serve a side of fruit at breakfast. Try to eat your fruit first and the rest of your meal second. As I've mentioned, fruit breaks down quickly in the body. If you eat a slow-digesting protein before fruit, the fruit will ferment in your intestine.

• Add a vegetable to every recipe. Before you eat anything, ask yourself, "Can I add a vegetable to this?" For instance, could you add lettuce to a sandwich, chopped broccoli to your eggs, or chopped veggies to pasta sauce or soup?

FILTERED WATER

STOP AGING PRESCRIPTION: 8 8-OUNCE GLASSES A DAY

The human body is 65 to 70 percent water by weight. Every cell—from the cells in your scalp to the cells in your toes—requires water to function. Water transports nutrients and oxygen to cells as well as removing waste products (acids). For this reason alone, water is critical to keeping body pH in balance.

Water is also the main component of blood, gastric juice, saliva, and urine. Without enough water, digestion does not run smoothly. You may already know this firsthand. Have you ever become dehydrated because you traveled on an airplane? Perhaps you purposely went without water in an attempt to avoid using the airplane bathroom. Or perhaps you just didn't manage to drink all that much during the hustle and bustle of traveling. Whatever the reason, you know all too well the price you paid—days and days of constipation.

Water also provides lubrication and shock protection to the body's joints, organs, and tissues. Adequate amounts of water also may go a long way to preventing dry and itchy skin, fatigue, and headaches. It may even reduce levels of the harmful stress hormone cortisol.

Make sure your water is pure. By pure, I mean water that does not contain harmful inorganic metals. If you drink municipal water or well water straight out of a tap, you probably are not drinking pure water. Some municipalities use the chemical monochloramine to disinfect drinking water supplies. Research done at the University of Missouri-Rolla has shown that this water-treatment technique can dissolve the lead in pipes, leaching it into the water. Few homes built after 1986 have lead pipes, but newer "lead-free" plumbing may, by law, contain up to 8 percent lead. Lead may also exist in service lines and other piping that leads to your home, in very small amounts in flow regulators, check valves, water meters, and brass faucets and fixtures.

If your municipality doesn't use monochloramine to disinfect drinking water, it almost definitely uses chlorine. This chemical reacts with organic matter in the water and is known to create by-products that are suspected carcinogens.

Well water, for various reasons, may not be completely safe, either. If you have hard water, then your well water can corrode your pipes, contaminating your water with any number of substances. Also, weed killers, pest killers, fertilizers, and other lawn chemicals can end up in well water. These products, even in minute amounts, are just as harmful when ingested by humans as they are when ingested by bugs. Finally, depending on the type of rock formations and soil surrounding your well, your water may be unusually high in flouride. In very low amounts, fluoride has been shown to improve dental health, but in high amounts it weakens teeth and bones.

Do you need to buy bottled water? While mineral and bottled waters are good, you don't need to forgo tap water. You just need a good water filter. Get one for your kitchen sink as well as for your shower head and bathroom sinks.

STOP AGING FACT

When are you more likely to become dehydrated: during the hot summer months or during the cold winter months? As it turns out, many people become dehydrated in the winter, rather than the summer. Why? During the summer, when we sweat a lot and generally feel hot, we feel thirstier, which reminds us to drink more fluids. In the winter, however, cold temperatures blunt this natural thirst mechanism by as much as 40 percent, according to studies done at the University of New Hampshire. Coldness causes the body to concentrate blood flow at the core, preventing the brain cells from sensing dehydration.

What if you are not a "water person"? I hear this quite often from my patients who prefer the taste of soda and other flavored beverages. I have good news: all of these patients—even the most adamant water haters—succeeded in increasing their water intake. If they can do it, so can you. Below, you will find some tips that have helped my patients and me.

• Make it festive. Once of my patients, Judy, finds she more easily meets her water intake if she drinks it from her prettiest champagne glass. The visual cue of the glass makes the experience feel special to her. Another patient likes to fill up a giant punch bowl with water along with sliced lemons and oranges for a festive touch. Throughout the day, she returns again and again to the bowl and refills her "punch" glass.

• Drink it at room temperature. Room-temperature water is easier to drink than ice water.

- Add a squeeze of lemon. The lemon juice will flavor the water, making it more enticing. Although lemon is acidic outside of the body, your stomach and intestines break it down into alkalinizing components during digestion.

- Drink a glass of water first thing in the morning. As soon as you roll out of bed, have your Alkalinizing Cocktail (which counts as one of your glasses of water), followed by a glass of water. I have found that when my patients and I consume water first thing, we feel thirstier during the day, which cues us to drink more water.

- Dilute your favorite beverage with water. As you wean yourself off soda and other sugary drinks, dilute them with water to increase your fluid intake. Eventually, you want to use no more than a shot glass full of a flavored beverage in each glass of water.

- Flavor it with juice or herbal tea. Try making a bunch of ice mint tea or putting just a tiny amount of juice in with your water.

GARLIC AND ONIONS

STOP AGING PRESCRIPTION: USE DAILY LIBERALLY

Garlic and onions are wonderful ways to spice up your meals. More important, these spices offer plenty of health benefits. In addition to their alkalinizing properties, both contain the phytochemical allicin, which has been shown to reduce the risk of certain types of cancer, lower blood cholesterol, and reduce blood pressure. This phyto-chemical also inhibits harmful bacteria, molds, and yeast. Research done at University Hospital Maastricht in the Netherlands, for example, has shown that garlic kills the ulcer-causing stomach bacterium *Helicobacter pylori*. Other research shows that garlic reduces the incidence of colds and flu, partly by killing these germs directly and partly by improving the function of the immune system.

Garlic and onions also help to fend off heart disease. Studies have found that the consumption of half a clove to a clove a day of garlic can reduce blood cholesterol levels by 10 percent.

In addition to allicin, garlic and onions contain quercetins, which reduce the severity of allergies, slow cancer growth, and protect the lungs from air pollution and other irritants. Finally, both garlic and onions feed beneficial bacteria in the gut, improving digestion. Both spices make frequent appearances in the Stop Aging recipes.

ALKALINIZING SPICES

STOP AGING PRESCRIPTION: USE SPICES LIBERALLY WHEN COOKING

Herbs and spices are a great way to flavor your food. The more delicious your food tastes, the more pleasurable neurochemical responses you generate in your brain. More important, herbs and spices allow you to flavor your food without the use of table salt, which is acid-producing. (Sea salt, as you'll soon learn, is alkalinizing.) Even better, nearly all herbs and spices help alkalinize the body. Many also contain potent disease-fighting antioxidants. Some of the disease-fighting powerhouses include chives, mint, basil, oregano, rosemary, sage, thyme, turmeric, ginger, licorice root, anise, caraway, celery, chervil, cilantro, cinnamon, coriander, cumin, dill, fennel, parsley, and tarragon.

FRUIT

STOP AGING PRESCRIPTION: USE FRUIT JUICE AND FRUIT PUREES IN PLACE OF SUGAR IN COOKING; EAT 2+ SERVINGS OF FRUIT A DAY

Like brightly colored vegetables, fruit offers many Stop Aging benefits. Most fruits alkalinize the body. They are also a rich source of many different vitamins that skin cells need for proper functioning. In particular, fruits are rich in vitamin C. They also house beta-carotene, which the body converts into vitamin A.

Fruits also contain lots and lots of water, which not only helps flush excess acid out of the body but also hydrates the skin. Most fruits contain digestion-promoting fiber, too, along with nutrients that feed beneficial gut bacteria.

STOP AGING FACT

Fruit tastes sweet because the trees and bushes that produce fruit *want* you to eat that fruit. The only way a plant can reproduce is by having animals eat its fruit and consequently spread that fruit's seeds. Fruit tastes sweetest when it is ripe, which, interestingly, is also when the fruit's seeds are biologically ready to take root.

Most fruits contain flavonoids that slow the production of harmful free radicals. In a study of elderly men completed in the Netherlands, study participants who consumed the most flavonoids reduced their risk of heart disease by 60 percent and stroke by 70 percent compared to participants who consumed the least amount of these protective substances.

LEMONS AND LIMES

STOP AGING PRESCRIPTION: SQUEEZE A WEDGE INTO AT LEAST TWO GLASSES OF WATER DAILY; USE LIBERALLY IN FOOD PREPARATION, PARTICULARLY TO FLAVOR SALADS

Although they are technically fruits, I've included a separate prescription for lemons and limes because they provide you with one of the most convenient ways to balance pH. Their sourness screams acidity to our taste buds, but lemons and limes powerfully alkalinize the body after digestion. For this reason alone, I recommend you drink lemon or lime water whenever you eat an acid-producing food such as beef. If you are out at a party, have a glass of lemon or lime water after every glass of wine or beer (or other alcoholic drink).

In addition to their alkalinizing effect, lemons and limes contain many different protective phytochemicals. Their flavonoids, for example, may help to halt tumor growth. Both lemons and limes inhibit harmful bacteria. Researchers from West Africa have found that lime juice kills off the bacteria that causes cholera. Finally, both contain high amounts of vitamin C, important in the production of collagen in the skin.

NUTS AND SEEDS

STOP AGING PRESCRIPTION: EAT THEM IN PLACE OF ACID-PRODUCING CRUNCHY SNACK FOODS

Most nuts and seeds are alkalinizing. This makes sense, as our ancient ancestors literally lived on them. Nuts contain a wealth of health-promoting nutrients, including monounsaturated fat, fiber, vitamin E, folic acid, copper, and magnesium. They also contain natural cholesterol-lowering substances called sterols, the same substances used in Benecol and other "cholesterol-lowering" margarines.

A study of eighty-six thousand nurses conducted at Brigham and Women's Hospital in Boston and the Harvard School of Public Health found that nurses who ate more than 5 ounces of nuts per week (the amount of nuts in a handful) had one-third fewer heart attacks than those who rarely or never ate nuts. Additional research has linked nut consumption with reduced cholesterol levels and a reduced risk of developing type 2 diabetes, macular degeneration (an eye disease that leads to blindness), and gallstones. Some researchers estimate that eating nuts regularly may lengthen your life by two years. Most are also high in fiber, which should help to improve digestion.

All of the health benefits aside, nuts and seeds taste fantastic. They offer a crunch that makes them the perfect snack food. Eat them instead of processed snack foods (chips, crackers, pretzels).

Note: Specific types of nuts and legumes such as peanuts, cashews, and pistachios may contain mold spores that could theoretically reduce levels of beneficial gut bacteria. If you experience a lot of gas and bloating, it's probably a good idea to avoid these specific varieties.

ALKALINIZING OILS

STOP AGING PRESCRIPTION: USE IT IN PLACE OF OTHER COOKING OILS
Olive, flaxseed, avocado, coconut, and macadamia oils all alkalinize the body. I recommend you experiment with all of them, as they lend slightly different tastes. Avocado is wonderful to put on your skin as well. For that reason, you'll find it in many of my skin care recipes in chapter 10.

In addition to alkalinizing the body, olive oil in particular offers many other youth-promoting benefits. Studies have shown that olive oil offers protection against heart disease by controlling LDL ("bad") cholesterol levels while raising HDL ("good") cholesterol levels. Olive oil is also a rich source of phytochemicals called polyphenols, which may be important in cancer prevention. Most of the Stop Aging recipes use olive oil, as it is the most affordable and available type of alkalinizing oil for food preparation. A few recipes use another oil—sesame or peanut—because in those cases the other oil contributes to a better-tasting end product.

ALKALINIZING WHOLE GRAINS

STOP AGING PRESCRIPTION: EAT OATS, WILD RICE, AND QUINOA IN PLACE OF OTHER GRAINS; USE OAT FLOUR WHENEVER POSSIBLE WHEN BAKING; LOOK FOR HIGH-FIBER BREAKFAST CEREALS MADE FROM OATS RATHER THAN WHEAT
Although there is some debate on the matter, most pH experts agree that wheat and rice acidify the body, whereas oats, quinoa, and wild rice (technically a grass and not a true rice) alkalinize the body. When you pair oats, quinoa, or wild rice with a large side of vegetables, you create the perfect alkalinizing accompaniment for any type of meat. These grains are also whole, which means they have not been refined. Because they include the entire grain, these foods contain healthful amounts of fiber, plant protein, and phytonutrients.

ASK DR. GRAF

Q: How is wild rice different from other types of rice?

A: Wild rice is actually not rice, but rather a grass with long grains. It's firmer and chewier than white or brown rice. The dark color you see in wild rice grains comes from health-promoting chlorophyll. Like other whole grains, wild rice is high in protein, the amino acid lysine, and fiber. It is also a good source of the minerals potassium and phosphorus, and the vitamins thiamine, riboflavin, and niacin.

SEA SALT

STOP AGING PRESCRIPTION: USE IT IN PLACE OF TABLE SALT
Sea salt alkalinizes the body, whereas table salt creates acids. You may rightly wonder: how can one salt be harmful while another is helpful? Isn't all salt the same? Not necessarily. All salt generally starts out roughly the same. Salt originates either from evaporated ocean water (sea salt) or from land salt deposits (rock salt). Depend-

ing on its origin, some natural salts contain more or less of certain types of trace minerals in addition to sodium chloride.

The main difference between table salt and sea salt, however, does not stem from its origin. Rather, it stems from how the salt was handled after it was taken from the ocean or the ground. First, let's take a look at table salt.

The salt in your salt shaker is *refined*. By that, I mean that it has been processed in such a way that nearly all of its natural trace minerals have been removed, creating a salt that is more than 95 percent sodium chloride. For this reason, table salt acidifies the body. It lacks natural minerals that would normally neutralize the acids sodium chloride creates. This processing, interestingly, was not done for nutritional purposes. About 93 percent of mined salt does not make it to your dinner table. Rather, it's used for industrial purposes, including manufacturing pulp and paper, setting dyes in textiles and fabric, and producing soaps and detergents. For these industrial uses, salt must be pure.

In addition to being stripped of its natural trace minerals, table salt also contains some additives that may or may not be all that good for your health. It contains anti-caking agents such as sodium silicoaluminate to ensure that the salt crystals more easily flow out of your shaker. It usually contains small amounts of sugar to prevent the salt from turning yellow when exposed to sunlight. Most table salts have also been fortified with iodine. Kosher salt is a step up from table salt, as it contains no preservatives. Some kosher salts are also sea salts, because they come from evaporated sea water. Others are rock salt.

Unlike table salt and kosher salt, sea salt contains many trace minerals important in neutralizing acids. Sea salt also remains in its original crystalline form. Some biophysicists have suggested that the crystalline structure of sea salt contains live energy. It vibrates with a frequency, and continues to vibrate as it mixes with the fluids of your body after consumption. No studies exist, however, to show that this vibrational quality matters to your good health.

Many people ask me whether they will become iodine-deficient if they forgo table salt for sea salt, which is not iodine-fortified. You need extremely small amounts of iodine for the proper functioning of your thyroid gland. Most Americans consume 700 micrograms of iodine a day, whereas they need less than 200 micrograms. In addition to table salt, you'll find iodine in bread, dairy products, most processed foods, seafood, and seaweed. Two or three servings of seafood a week give you all the natural iodine you need.

ASK DR. GRAF

Q: I have high blood pressure. Shouldn't I limit salt?

A: I'm not asking you to add more salt to your diet. Rather, I'm suggesting that you use sea salt in place of table salt. Doing so should help you to naturally reduce your overall salt intake. A teaspoon of table salt contains more sodium (because of its very fine grains) than a tablespoon of coarse sea salt (because of its larger grains). The Stop Aging menus will also naturally help you to reduce your sodium consumption by encouraging you to eat fewer sodium-rich processed foods and more mineral-rich fruits and vegetables. I think you'll be pleasantly surprised to see your blood pressure going *down* once you switch to Stop Aging eating. To stay on the safe side, however, do monitor your blood pressure closely as you make this dietary change, and definitely run it by your doctor.

Acid-Producing Age Accelerators

Minimize the following foods as much as possible. Whenever you consume an acid-producing food, balance that consumption by pairing it with an Age Stopper food.

SUGAR

STOP AGING PRESCRIPTION: DO NOT USE TABLE SUGAR; CUT BACK ON ADDED SUGARS FROM PROCESSED FOODS AS MUCH AS POSSIBLE

Sugar is bug juice. Place some jelly on a plate outdoors and what happens? It attracts flies and other bugs. Dissolve a pinch of sugar in a cup of warm water and add some yeast and what happens? The yeast multiply into a froth.

The same thing happens inside your body. As I mentioned in

chapter 3, your GI tract contains millions of bacteria, yeast, and other organisms. Sugar feeds harmful gut organisms, especially yeast. When you eat sugar, yeast overgrows, crowding out beneficial bacteria and creating toxic by-products. These days I see more patients with toenail fungus, dandruff, and athlete's foot than ever before. Quite often when I ask them about their nutritional habits, I learn that they eat quite a bit of sugar.

Sugar also makes you more susceptible to infection. Eating or drinking 8 tablespoons of sugar (the equivalent of two and a half 12-ounce cans of soda) has been shown to reduce the ability of white blood cells to kill germs by as much as 40 percent. This effect starts within thirty minutes of ingestion and may last as long as five hours.

High intakes of sugar have been linked to obesity, heart disease, tooth decay, diabetes, and premature aging. Some types of sugar chemically alter proteins, creating advanced glycosylation end products (AGEs) that collect in various tissues, inhibiting their function. In the skin, this results in a loss of elasticity (sagging, wrinkling).

I recommend you eliminate as much refined sugar from your diet as possible. To do so, consider this advice:

• Use 100 percent fruit juice and or molasses to sweeten baked goods, using these alkalinizing sweeteners in place of some or all of the sugar in a recipe.

• Cut back on the sugar in your recipes. You can probably eliminate as much as half of the sugar in a dessert recipe and still enjoy the finished product.

• Add alkalinizing ingredients to sweet baked goods whenever possible. Consider adding oatmeal to your chocolate chip cookie recipe, for example.

• Read labels carefully. Try not to purchase foods that list sugar, high-fructose corn syrup, corn syrup, or evaporated cane juice among the first three ingredients.

• Develop a fruit tooth. Berries, kiwi, and other types of fruit are nature's original sweet desserts. Packed with health-promoting antioxidants, plant pigments, and fiber, fruit will help turn down your sugar cravings and appetite.

PROCESSED CARBOHYDRATES

STOP AGING PRESCRIPTION: EAT "REAL" FOOD AS OFTEN AS POSSIBLE

Processed carbohydrates start out as plants: corn chips come from corn, flour comes from wheat. Yet most of the high-carbohydrate foods you see lining the shelves of your grocery store don't look like plants. Indeed, they've been chopped, ground, hulled, and otherwise changed from their original state. Whatever beneficial plant nutrients that existed in their original forms are gone by the time these refined grains make their way into most crackers, chips, and other processed foods. What's left? A starchy, sugary, empty-calorie, fiberless product. It's no surprise that a diet rich in sugar and processed foods has been linked with high blood sugar, heart disease, and constipation.

I have another problem with processed foods. Unlike fruits, vegetables, and seeds, processed foods are dead. Because they contain no live enzymes, they don't change in structure as they sit on a shelf. If you stop to think about it, you'll agree with me that there's something inherently wrong with a food that doesn't spoil. If a food can still be eaten a year or more after its creation, can it really be good for you? I don't think so. I can't cite a study for you, but I'm willing to place a big wager that the longer a food's shelf life, the more that food shortens your life span.

I'd like you to put processed carbohydrate foods in the same mental category that you do sugar. They act the same way in the body. They are merely empty sources of calories, and they have no place on your Stop Aging plate.

Use these pointers to reduce your consumption of processed foods:

• Whenever possible, choose foods made from the Stop Aging power grains oatmeal, quinoa, or wild rice. These are the only grains that alkalinize the body.

• When choosing foods made from other grains, look for products labeled as "100 percent whole grain." Whole-grain products contain some or all of the original goodness of the grain. They may be acid-producing in the body, but they also supply you with digestion-optimizing fiber and health-promoting phytonutrients.

ALCOHOL

STOP AGING PRESCRIPTION: NO MORE THAN ONE TO TWO DRINKS A DAY

Many types of alcohol contain health-promoting phytochemicals, so it's not surprising that studies have linked moderate consumption of alcohol with good health. For example, moderate consumption of alcohol has been associated with a reduced incidence of heart disease and stroke.

So why is alcohol on the Age Accelerator list? Because alcohol is also extremely acid-producing in the body. When the liver breaks down ethanol, it strips it of its electrons, creating acetic acid. This is the same very-low-pH acid found in vinegar. Perhaps because it dramatically lowers pH, alcohol reduces the effectiveness of your white blood cells. This is why you catch colds so easily after a night of heavy drinking. Also, because 20 percent of the alcohol you drink gets absorbed through the stomach wall rather than the intestine, alcohol may increase your risk of stomach ulcers.

STOP AGING FACT

Many people turn to the bottle in order to forget a bad experience. Interestingly, research shows that drinking may actually reinforce bad memories, causing them to stay with you longer. Ohio State University researchers have found in animal studies that moderate drinking—the human equivalent of two drinks a day—improves memory of both positive and negative events. Alcohol does this by increasing the expression of a receptor on the surface of brain cells. "People who drink to forget bad memories may actually be doing the opposite by reinforcing the neural circuits that control negative emotional memory," wrote study author Matthew During, a professor of virology, immunology, and cancer genetics. By the way, although excessive drinking (six or seven drinks a day) temporarily increased memory, it also damaged brain cells, which would eventually reduce memory over time.

I love sipping a glass of red wine at night, so I'm not going to suggest you give up alcohol if you enjoy it. Instead, use this advice:

- Have no more than two alcoholic drinks a day.
- Consume a glass of lemon or lime water before or after each alcoholic drink.
- The morning after drinking alcohol (especially if you are feeling hung over) put an extra scoop of greens powder in your Alkalinizing Cocktail (you'll learn more about how to make this important drink in the next chapter).

COLAS

STOP AGING PRESCRIPTION: GIVE THEM UP

Cola is probably the worst beverage you can drink. A typical 12-ounce can of cola contains 44 to 62 milligrams of phosphoric acid. This phosphoric acid comes in a package that usually also includes other acid-producing substances (sugar and caffeine) and absolutely no minerals (such as calcium or potassium) to buffer the acids that it creates. As a result, the phosphorus binds with any dietary calcium you consume from other foods, preventing the calcium from being absorbed.

When researchers at the Naval Medical Research Institute placed human teeth in a cola beverage, the phosphoric acid softened and dissolved the teeth! The same happens to the bones inside your body. In a Harvard study of 1,672 women and 1,148 men, participants who drank cola daily had more reduced bone mineral density than participants who drank cola once a week or less often.

Loss of body calcium does more than weaken bones. It interferes with cell signaling. In short, when you drink too much cola, your blood, bones, and cells don't have enough calcium to function optimally. Not only does this contribute to poor skin health, it also raises your risk of heart disease, colon cancer, and osteoporosis. What is the only guaranteed way to avoid the acid-producing effects of cola? Don't drink it!

I realize that it's not going to be easy to break your cola-drinking habit. Try these tips:

- If you need something sweet to drink, try 100 percent, no-sugar-added fruit juice. It's alkalinizing and provides your body with health-promoting phytochemicals. I also strongly recommend you purchase a juicer. It will allow you to make your own signature fruit juices, altering flavors as needed to suit your personal tastes.

- If you are not a water person, try seltzer or club soda. For more taste, add a splash of fruit juice or a squeeze of lemon or lime.

- If you need the caffeine, try green tea. It's alkalinizing, contains caffeine to keep you awake, and also supplies your body with health-promoting phytochemicals. Some components in green tea may even speed metabolism, helping you to lose weight if that is one of your goals.

COFFEE

STOP AGING PRESCRIPTION: CUT BACK, AND SWITCH TO VARIETIES THAT PRODUCE LESS ACID

Since I'm an avid coffee fan, it's with much regret that I inform you that coffee is acid-producing. In addition to acidifying the body, the 135 milligrams of caffeine in each 8-ounce cup of brewed coffee elevate circulating levels of epinephrine, which increases your overall stress level. That's strike two. Now for strike three. Both caffeinated coffee and decaffeinated coffee increase the production of stomach acid as well as prevent the proper closure of the valve between the stomach and esophagus, leading to heartburn.

With the bad news, however, also comes some good. Coffee is one of nature's laxatives, so it may help improve digestive health. Studies have also linked coffee consumption with a reduced incidence of gallstones, improved blood sugar levels, and a reduced risk of liver and colon cancer and of Parkinson's disease. Why? Like other plant foods—and coffee does come from a plant—coffee is a rich source of antioxidant phytochemicals called polyphenols. Due to the low intakes of fruits and vegetables in this country, coffee is actually the number one source of antioxidants in the U.S. diet!

Here's what I suggest you do to balance the good and the bad:

- Hold yourself to about 200 milligrams of caffeine, the amount in two 8-ounce cups of brewed coffee or two shots of espresso.

Research shows that this level of caffeine lifts mood and energy. Once you go above 200 milligrams, however, you'll start to notice negative side effects such as jitteriness, anxiety, and stomach upset.

• Consider choosing coffee made from the arabica bean, which has about half the amount of caffeine as the robusta bean, the other main variety.

• Drink less coffee if you take birth control pills. It takes longer to metabolize caffeine when you're on the pill.

• To prevent withdrawal symptoms as you cut back, replace some of the coffee you drink with green tea, which is alkalinizing. Green tea also blocks the growth of harmful gut bacteria.

• Get the acid out of your coffee. Drink only freshly brewed organic coffee made from freshly ground beans. Acids build up in ground coffee over time and especially in brewed coffee that has been sitting on a warming plate.

ANIMAL PROTEIN

STOP AGING PRESCRIPTION: NO MORE THAN 8 OUNCES OF MEAT OR DAIRY EACH DAY

As I mentioned, all protein—whether it comes from an animal or a plant—creates acids in the body. Most plant proteins, however, come complete with alkalinizing components—particularly potassium—that neutralize any acids their proteins create. Animal protein does not come in this pH-balanced package, making it universally acid-producing.

Many studies have linked overconsumption of animal protein (and the resulting increase in body uric acid) with a host of different diseases. Research completed at the University of Texas Southwestern Medical Center in Dallas found that switching from a balanced diet to a high-protein, low-carbohydrate diet raised acid excretion in the kidneys by 90 percent (an indication of increased acid production in the body). At the same time, the switch to a high-protein regimen reduced citrate (an alkalinizing substance that prevents kidney stones) by 25 percent. This type of acid load has been known to increase the incidence of kidney stones and cause a drop in bone mass.

You don't have to give up protein to stop aging. You need only eat it in balance with alkalinizing foods. No more than 10 to 15 percent of your calories should come from animal protein (including protein from dairy). For most people, that's no more than 8 ounces of meat daily.

When you eat meat, choose the healthiest varieties possible to counterbalance the acids that meats naturally create. To do so, follow these pointers:

• Choose organic varieties whenever possible. Conventionally raised chicken and livestock are routinely dosed with antibiotics to prevent them from getting infections (which are usually caused by living in close quarters, eating grain instead of a natural diet, and hormone injections). Small amounts of these antibiotics may remain in the meat after slaughter and could theoretically kill off some beneficial bacteria in your gut when you eat these foods.

Conventionally raised meat—especially beef—is treated with hormones to promote growth. These hormones make their way into the meat. A Harvard study of more than ninety thousand women found that consumption of red meat was associated with a specific type of hormone-dependent breast cancer.

STOP AGING TIP

If you could pick the cow or pig that produced the meat you ate, I'm making an educated guess that you would choose the healthiest animal. You'd probably refuse to eat meat from a cow that appeared sick or diseased. Unfortunately, you probably do not have the option of picking your meat source before slaughter, but you can still get a good idea of the health of the animal that produced the meat. Just go by the color of the meat. Low pH is just as bad for livestock as it is for humans. As it turns out, excess acids damage muscle proteins in animals, causing the meat they produce to appear pale and watery. So when choosing meat at the store, choose the darker, richer-colored options (assuming you are comparing like cuts). By the way, meat that is more alkaline generally tastes better, too, so you'll be doing both your body and your taste buds a favor.

• Look for grass-fed beef over grain-fed varieties. Grass-fed beef contains slightly more beneficial omega-3 fatty acids than grain-fed beef. These fatty acids are important for brain health, skin health, and immunity.

• Allow a good amount of your animal protein consumption to come from organic eggs. Eggs are a complete food that contain all the amino acids needed for life. They are also a rich source of linoleic acid (a polyunsaturated fat), minerals, most B vitamins, and the anti-oxidants lutein and zeaxanthin. Eggs almost compare with plants in terms of the nutrition they provide.

• Load up on alkalinizing foods whenever you eat meat. Let's say you want to have a steak. Go ahead and enjoy one. Just balance it by starting your meal with a large salad. Then accompany your steak with just as large a serving of sautéed greens or steamed vegetables and an alkalinizing starch or grain such as wild rice or sweet potato.

ASK DR. GRAF

Q: Won't my bones weaken if I don't drink three glasses of milk a day?

A: Chinese and Japanese women have lower fracture rates than American women, despite the fact that they drink little to no milk. Although dairy products do indeed contain high amounts of bone-building calcium, they also contain acid-producing protein. A high intake of animal protein — including milk protein — causes the body to excrete calcium in the urine. Dairy products simply are not the best way to get calcium to your bones.

Balancing your pH will go a long way toward strengthening your bones. Also, the Stop Aging menus are rich in kale, collards, and other dark leafy greens that are all excellent sources of calcium. In addition to calcium, other vitamins and minerals are important to bone health. They include vitamin C, magnesium, potassium, and zinc. Components in tea and onions seem to slow the loss of bone as well, even though these foods do not contain calcium.

Indulge Without Guilt

Okay, so now you are armed with the knowledge you need to switch over to Stop Aging eating. Life change, however, is about more than just knowledge. It's also about motivation. So let me leave you with the following pep talk.

You may wonder, as you go through the effort of changing your diet, whether it's truly worth it. Will all of these changes really add up to a more youthful you? I'd like you to trust me, but I'll go one better—I'll give you a study to trust instead. Researchers in Australia studied the diets of people living in Australia, Sweden, and Greece. They found that people who ate a diet rich in dark leafy greens (an Age Stopper food), vegetables (another Age Stopper), olive oil (yet another Age Stopper), and nuts (a fourth Age Stopper), minimizing red meat (an Age Accelerator) and sugar (another Age Accelerator), had fewer wrinkles than people who ate more of the Age Accelerators and fewer of the Age Stoppers.

Also, it's important to know that while cutting back on Age Accelerators may be hard at first, it won't always feel so difficult. As you progress on the Stop Aging, Start Living Plan, weaning yourself off sugar and other acid-producing foods will become easier and easier. You simply won't want them! As you balance pH, you'll lose some of your affinity for sugar, cola, red meat, and other foods. Your taste preferences will change. You'll find that you naturally prefer alkalinizing foods over acid-producing ones.

6

the stop aging supplement prescription

You won't be taking many supplements on this plan. As I've mentioned, I don't believe in spending lots of money on many different supplements or in gulping down pill after pill. For that reason, I require only three daily Stop Aging supplements. The supplements I've prescribed in this chapter provide you with the nutritional insurance policy to counteract your guilty pleasures (red meat, sugar, caffeine, wine), fill nutritional gaps in your daily diet, and overcome the shortcomings of the modern food supply.

In a perfect world, you wouldn't need any supplements. Unfortunately, we don't live in a perfect world, and our food supply isn't as nutritious as it used to be. Even if you managed to eat perfectly every single day—never allowing your acid-producing foods to outnumber your alkalinizing foods—you would still need a few supplements.

Acid-producing farming practices (especially the use of commercial fertilizers) and acid rain have demineralized our soils. As a result, today's produce does not contain as many minerals as produce that grew just half a century ago. According to one study, today's carrots have 75 percent less magnesium, 48 percent less calcium, 46 percent less iron, and 75 percent less copper than carrots grown fifty years ago. Conventionally grown carrots have even fewer minerals than organically grown varieties.

Few of us eat as healthfully as we should. I definitely have my good days and my not-so-good days when it comes to eating. I have days when I'm running from appointment to appointment and handling one crisis after another. On those days, I rarely eat as many vegetables as I'd like. I also am not willing to give up some cherished acid-producing foods. I love coffee. I love wine. To balance these loves, I'd have to eat far more greens and vegetables than I could ever find time to prepare. It's for these reasons that I began researching supplements, and why I recommend the same supplements to you.

Recommended Supplements

The supplements I recommend in the sections that follow are no more than food in a pill. I feel confident that they are safe for everyone, but it's always a good idea to check with your doctor before taking any supplement, especially if you are taking prescription medications.

THE ALKALINIZING COCKTAIL

STOP AGING PRESCRIPTION: 1+ TIMES A DAY

The Alkalinizing Cocktail is the cornerstone of the Stop Aging, Start Living Plan. If you don't have the motivation, time, or energy to change your diet, then at least drink the cocktail each morning. It will fuel you with the energy you need to change the way you eat.

The cocktail is a combination of the following two powdered supplements: powdered greens and powdered fiber, with extra spirulina (a type of powdered algae) thrown in as an option. Although it may not sound very appealing, trust me—the thought of drinking it is much worse than the actual experience. Assuming you purchase the brands I recommend and make your cocktail as directed, it actually tastes sweet, goes down easily, and, most important, makes you feel incredible.

I stumbled across the greens powder many years ago, after that juice fast that I mentioned earlier. I knew I needed more fruits and vegetables in my diet, but I was constantly on the move, going from patient to patient. I traveled frequently. Sometimes—often with the help of my juicer—I managed to eat ten servings of fruits and vegetables in a given day. Usually I did not, especially when I traveled. As committed as I was to juicing, I wasn't willing to lug the juicer with me on an airplane.

So I began looking for a more concentrated and convenient source of fruits and vegetables. I discovered greens powders. Sold online and in health food stores, greens powders are nothing fancier than a powdered form of vegetable juice. You mix the powder with water and drink. Most notably, these powders are rich sources of wheat and barley grasses, sprouted grains, broccoli, kale, and other green vegetables. Wheat, barley, and other cereal grasses in particular are extremely rich in antioxidants, chlorophyll, protein, vitamins, and minerals. The grasses—the youngest green sprouts of these cereal grains—are actually much more nutritious than the grains (wheat, barley, kamut) that they produce. They are particularly rich in polyphenols, the colorful pigments in fruits and vegetables that have been shown to promote optimal health.

Thanks to the nutritional goodness of these grasses, some greens drinks—such as my favorite brand, Greens First—contain antioxidant power equivalent to eating ten servings of fruits and vegetables! That's what I call concentrated nutrition.

I'll be honest with you. I've tried many different greens powders, and most of them are the equivalent of drinking pond scum. They don't dissolve well in water, creating a chalky, clumpy consistency. They taste even worse than they look. Many of the greens powders I've tried have actually caused me to gag. The only way I could get them down was to mix them with peach iced tea, pinch my nose, and chug.

It took two years before I found a greens powder that I liked and actually looked forward to drinking. I don't need to mix Greens First with juice or peach iced tea. It's perfect as is. The brand Greens+ runs a close second.

Greens powder is the most important component of your alkalinizing cocktail. In addition to the powder, you will also add the following ingredients.

Fiber. I suggest you mix a scoop or two of fiber into your cocktail. The fiber, as I've mentioned, will help improve digestion as well as improve pH. Fiber acts like a sponge, soaking up acids and toxins from the intestines. Health experts recommend you consume 25 to 30 grams of fiber a day, but most people consume 15 grams or fewer. How do you know if you're getting enough fiber? That's an easy one. How often and easily do you have bowel movements? If you easily have a bowel movement once a day, you're probably getting enough fiber. If you have small, hard-to-pass stool, you need more fiber and water.

My personal favorites are brands that are easily found in your local supermarket or drugstore. Benefiber and Fiber-sure are fiber in the form of a fine powder that easily dissolves into any liquid, including cereals, soups, drinks, and, most important, your Alkalinizing Cocktail. They do not add any grit or change the texture or taste of the cocktail, allowing the cocktail to go down smoothly. They are also available in small travel packets.

Alternatively, you could take a separate fiber supplement. I personally find it most convenient to mix it into the drink, as you need to drink a glass of water with most fiber supplements anyway.

Spirulina (optional). Spirulina is a type of blue-green algae found in most lakes and ponds. It is a rich source of amino acids, B complex vitamins, beta-carotene, vitamin E, carotenoids, manganese, zinc, copper, iron, selenium, and gamma-linolenic acid (an essential fatty acid). Because of its wealth of minerals, spirulina is exceptionally alkalinizing.

It also bolsters immunity. Animal and test tube studies have shown that spirulina increases production of cells that improve immunity and fight cancer. It also improves digestion by supporting the growth of beneficial bacteria in the gut.

It really is a wonderful supplement, but I've made it optional for one important reason: it tastes terrible. I've yet to find a powdered form of spirulina that doesn't ruin the taste of the Alkalinizing Cocktail. In lieu of putting it in your drink, you can also try spirulina in supplement form. Take 4 to 6 500 milligram capsules a day, for a total of 2,000 to 3,000 milligrams daily.

Alkaline fruit juices (optional). To improve the taste of your cocktail, you may choose any 100 percent fruit juice (no sugar added) of your liking, as nearly all of them are alkalinizing. Give yourself bonus points for pulling out the juicer and making your own fresh apple, pineapple, or other juice (see the juice recipes on pages 204–205).

Alkalinizing Cocktail Recipe

1 to 2 scoops greens powder

1 to 2 scoops fiber powder

1 tablespoon spirulina (optional)

100 percent fresh fruit juice (to taste and optional)

8 to 24 ounces of water (to desired consistency)

Place all ingredients in a shaker bottle with a tightly fitting lid. Shake vigorously for 10 to 15 seconds. Remove lid and drink.

MINERAL SUPPLEMENT WITH CALCIUM

STOP AGING PRESCRIPTION: ONE 500-MILLIGRAM SUPPLEMENT TWICE DAILY

Because alkalinizing minerals—calcium, potassium, and magnesium in particular—are so important, I recommend you also take a mineral supplement every day. As I've mentioned, minerals help to neutralize the acids created by protein, sugar, and other acid producing foods. If you don't consume enough minerals, your body will rob them from your bones and muscles.

You might be able to consume enough minerals naturally through food alone, but you have many different factors working against you. As I've mentioned, produce does not contain as many minerals as it used to. On top of that, you probably absorb fewer minerals from your food now than you did twenty years ago, or even five years ago. As we age, our stomachs become less efficient at producing stomach acid. Certain medications can also reduce stomach acid levels. You need stomach acid to break down calcium into a form that can be absorbed. A lower amount of acid hinders calcium absorption.

Of all the supplemental minerals, calcium is perhaps the most important. Almost every cell in the body, including those in the heart, nerves, and muscles, need calcium to function properly.

When you're looking for a supplement, choose one that contains calcium along with a mixture of other minerals such as potassium and magnesium. Check to see that the supplement contains more than one form of calcium. Supplement companies get calcium from many different sources. Try not to be swayed by marketing claims that tell you that they have used the form of calcium that is best absorbed in the intestine. There are differing benefits for every type of calcium. For instance, calcium carbonate isn't as well absorbed as calcium citrate, but calcium citrate is not as beneficial for colon health as calcium carbonate. Look for a supplement that contains both calcium carbonate and calcium citrate, and possibly other types of calcium as well, such as calcium malate, calcium lactate, or calcium gluconate.

Your supplement should contain only about 500 to 600 milligrams of calcium per pill, as this is the maximum amount your body can absorb at one time. Take one of these supplements twice a day. Try to take your mineral supplement at a different time of day than you have your greens drink, especially if you have fiber in the drink. Fiber speeds up stool transit time, preventing some of the calcium from being absorbed.

Probiotic Bacteria

STOP AGING PRESCRIPTION: 5 BILLION CFUS (COLONY-FORMING UNITS) DAILY

As I mentioned in chapter 3, healthy levels of certain types of gut bacteria can influence skin health in a number of ways. Most notably, these bacteria help to improve immunity, which in turn reduces the incidence of immune-related skin disorders such as dermatitis, psoriasis, and even acne.

Good bacteria also help to keep levels of bad bacteria and yeast in check. Yeast and some types of bacteria produce acids when they metabolize certain foods in the gut. As a result, high levels of good bacteria help to ensure that harmful gut organisms do not disrupt your pH.

The Stop Aging menus will help to improve digestion, but you need probiotics, too. I don't know too many people who are willing or able to completely give up all forms of sugar and completely ban nonorganic meat. Many gastrointestinal experts believe that our modern diets continually reduce levels of good gut bacteria, making daily supplementation a must.

> **STOP AGING TIP**
> Take your supplement on an empty stomach, but plan to eat fruit soon afterward. The fruit will help to feed the beneficial bacteria once it arrives in the colon, increasing the likelihood that it will stick around and multiply.

When shopping for a probiotic supplement, follow this advice:

• Don't worry too much about the long, hard-to-spell names of bacteria and yeast on these supplements. At this point, scientists don't know precisely which of these organisms are most beneficial, so rather than looking for one type in particular, look for a supplement that contains a mixture of different types.

• Gastric acids in the stomach and bile salts in the intestines kill off as many as 80 percent of the beneficial bacteria in your supplement, so you need to swallow *a lot* of it to ensure enough makes it through the stomach and into your intestines. Choose a supplement that contains at least 5 billion units (sometimes referred to as colony-forming units, or CFUs) per day.

• In a test of available probiotic supplements, the independent supplement testing company ConsumerLab.com found that eight of the twenty-two products tested contained less than 1 percent of the claimed number of live bacteria. Six products had only a few thousand live bacteria, much less than the 5 billion or so that you need. Consult the appendix for a list of brands that passed their test and contain the amount of bacteria claimed on the product labeling.

• Choose a refrigerated product. Exposure to heat, moisture, and oxygen can kill the bacteria organisms in a supplement.

• Check the expiration date. Bacteria will not live in a supplement for an eternity. If a product is past its date, don't buy it.

• Don't always assume enteric-coated supplements are superior. Some bacteria are better able to survive stomach acid than others. *Lactobacillus, Bifidobacterium,* and *Streptococcus* species do not need enteric coating, but *L. bulgaricus* and *S. thermophilus,* as well as *Leuconostoc* and *Lactococcus* species, do.

7

the stop aging
lifestyle prescription

The Stop Aging Lifestyle Prescription is the solution to a distressing life. You've already learned the importance of halting your stress response and turning on your relaxation response. All of the prescriptions in this chapter will help you do just that. They will also heighten the production of joy-producing neuropeptides that are so critical to bright, glowing skin.

These lifestyle prescriptions will help you to feel as good as they help you to look. Practice them regularly and you'll have more energy, feel less anxious, and generally feel happy and calm. Good health and beautiful skin never felt so decadent!

Fun Activity

STOP AGING PRESCRIPTION: ONE OR TWO TIMES A WEEK

With lives consumed by work, responsibilities, and lots of stress, many of us have forgotten what it feels like to laugh heartily and smile contagiously. As I mentioned in chapter 4, I realized a few years ago that something was seriously wrong with my life. I realized that I needed to have more fun, but it took me a few weeks to figure out *how*.

Dancing is my fun activity, but it may not be yours. I'm not recommending that you start dancing to improve your skin health. I *am* recommending that you get in touch with what drives you, what invigorates you, what makes you want to jump out of bed in the morning. Regular doses of fun will bring your life to the next level, raising it from good to great. Your fun activity will fill you with joy and other positive emotions that generate a glow that can't be replicated by any office procedure. Plus, smiling is the single best way to prevent frown lines!

A fun activity isn't something you watch—it doesn't consist of sitting in front of the television, attending a baseball game, or drinking cosmopolitans with your girlfriends. Your fun activity involves participating. You don't watch. You do.

Your fun activity is also unique to you. Your fun activity may be someone else's nightmare. Case in point: some of my patients *love* to run. They get up at 5:00 A.M. to *run*. They excitedly tell me about races, running routes, running times, and running partners. They gush about runner's high. Well, that's great—I'm happy for them. I'm glad they get their runner's high. For me, running is anything but fun. Rather than runner's high, I get runner's low.

To come up with your fun activity, consider these questions:

What activity makes you uniquely you?
What makes you want to get out of bed in the morning?
What made you laugh as a child?
What activities did you love as a child?
What do you consider fun?

Here I've listed some ideas to help get your thoughts flowing.

Creative expression. Painting, sculpting, drawing, even scrapbooking can count as your fun activity if you are the type of person who looks forward to expressing yourself creatively. Consider signing up for an art class. Or be less formal, by taking out some crayons, Magic Markers, or even Play-Doh. Think of how much fun you had as a child when you finger-painted, used watercolors, or sponge-painted. Try to rediscover that creativity and joy of expressing yourself in color and texture.

Connect with the earth. Some people feel exhilarated when they are outdoors. If the smells, sights, and sounds of nature get you out of bed in the morning, then consider taking up hiking, gardening, or walking on the beach.

Move it. What type of movement makes you feel good? Belly dancing? Yoga? Tai chi? Strip aerobics? It feels tantalizingly good to move the body in a way you don't generally move day in and day out. Don't automatically assume that movement can be fun only if you already know how to do it. When you must focus on coordinating and learning new movement patterns, you don't have the mental space to think about what you need to finish at the office. So be daring. Try something new. You may find it exhilarating.

As long as you love it and look forward to it, any type of movement can count. As an added bonus, a move-it fun activity can double as your exercise and may even triple as your relaxation! If you take up yoga, you may even be able to quadruple-task, getting your deep breathing activity in as well.

Music. Your fun activity may center on musical expression, whether it's singing or playing an instrument. If you are not musically trained, you might consider a drumming group. If you have small children, you might sign up for a Mommy and Me music class. Just make sure this is something that exhilarates you. It should not become just one more thing on your to-do list.

Play. Go to a playground and what do you see and hear? You probably don't see too many frowns or hear too much crying or whining, and if you do, it doesn't last for long. Indeed, children on a playground can teach you a great deal about having fun. If you're a parent, play with your children. Go down the slides. Swing. Climb the jungle gym. Play king of the mountain. Build sandcastles. It will bring you closer to your children, make you the most fun parent on the block, reduce stress, and help you look forward to each day with your family.

The idea for your fun activity might not come to you today. It might take a few weeks before something surfaces. You also may need to go through a few trial runs. For example, you might pick hiking as a fun activity, try it a few times, and then realize that you dread it. Again, if your fun activity becomes a stressor rather than a stress reliever, you need a new fun activity!

Once you've defined what's fun for you, schedule it in. Put it in your calendar, datebook, or personal organizer. Even though this is something that defines you and brings you great joy, you need to plan for it. Otherwise, it just won't happen. You'll start each day thinking that you might have time for some fun, but you won't make time. If you put it in your schedule, you'll have fun.

Also consider doing your fun activity with at least one other person. If you like to dance, consider periodically going to a line-dancing night or taking a ballroom or swing class. If you enjoy music, consider joining a band or singing group. If you love to move, run or ride a bike with a buddy. Social connections heighten the joy of the experience and will keep you coming back for more.

EXERCISE

STOP AGING PRESCRIPTION: TWENTY MINUTES OR MORE, FOUR TIMES A WEEK
Exercise probably slows the aging process in every part of your body. Not only does it strengthen your muscles, bones, heart, and lungs, it also helps prevent heart disease, diabetes, and certain types of cancer. And it helps you maintain a healthy weight.

Exercise improves blood circulation, which allows skin cells to receive nutrients and release wastes more easily. Perspiration during exercise helps you to balance body pH by pushing toxins and acids to the skin surface, where they evaporate. This directly translates into a youthful, glowing skin. It also may help reduce acne and allergic skin conditions that are caused in part by the buildup of acids and metabolic waste.

Perhaps most important, regular exercise seems to counteract photoaging of the skin. In a study completed at Rutgers University, researchers exposed rats to high amounts of ultraviolet light for fourteen weeks. During this time, half of the rats had access to an exercise wheel, whereas the other rats did not. After fourteen weeks of nearly constant sunlight exposure, the rats that ran on their wheels had 32 percent fewer skin cancer tumors than rats who did not exercise.

Exercise can also improve skin health by improving your mental outlook. Each time you exercise, you stimulate the release of endorphin peptides in the brain. These chemicals are the body's natural painkillers and can lead to an increase in feelings of happiness. Researchers at Duke University found that 60 percent of depressed study participants who exercised for thirty minutes three times a week overcame their depression without using antidepressant medication. Another study found that short workouts of eight minutes in length could help lower sadness, tension, and anger. Exercise also seems to improve confidence.

I know when I get into a downward slump of not exercising, I move into a different, more negative level of being. I feel sluggish and irritable, and I don't laugh as spontaneously or crack as many jokes.

While the Stop Aging Exercise Prescription—twenty minutes of exercise four times a week—is the ideal, keep in mind that this goal may not be right for you today, especially if you are currently out of shape. Too much exercise can be as destructive as too little. When you overtrain, your muscles generate more acid waste products than your circulatory system can clear. This results in soreness, fatigue, and irritability. Exercise should make you feel good. If it makes you feel bad, you're overdoing it.

Start slow. The ideal amount of exercise for you today may be five minutes. Next month it may be ten.

Also, trust that exercise will become easier over time. It may feel hard in the beginning because you are getting used to something new. It may feel awkward or frustrating. During the getting-in-shape stage, when you don't know what your body can really handle, you may have a tendency to overdo it, feeling the next morning as if you just went twelve rounds with a heavyweight boxer. This stage does not last long. Usually after just a couple of weeks, most of the post-exercise soreness subsides as your body gets used to the movement.

Here is some advice for starting and maintaining an exercise plan:

• Do it while surrounded by beauty. A wooded trail, striking vista, or ocean scene will add to the endorphins already being stimulated by the movement. You'll have true bliss.

• Make it mindful. Periodically bring your attention inward. If you are walking, notice how it feels as each foot hits the ground. If you are swimming, concentrate on the sensation of water streaming over your body. If you are dancing, feel how your muscles move.

This again will enhance that mind-body connection, allowing those endorphins to flood you with joy.

• Think of it as a gift. Rather than thinking of exercise as punishment—something you have to do to look and feel better—change your focus. Consider exercise a gift that you give yourself. It's a respite of quiet time when you don't need to achieve or strive.

DEEP BREATHING

STOP AGING PRESCRIPTION: FIVE MINUTES TWICE A DAY

I'd like you to try something. Get a watch or a timer, put this book down, and count how many times you breathe in a minute. Go do it, and then come back to the book when you are done.

How many breaths did you take? Twelve? Fifteen? Twenty? If so, know that you are *very* normal. Most people breathe twelve to fifteen times a minute. Yet in this case, normal isn't ideal.

This rapid breathing rate is out of sync with the natural rhythms of the body. Your heartbeat, blood vessels, and brain waves operate on a set rhythm, known as the *Mayer wave frequency,* that aligns with an ideal breathing rate of six breaths a minute. Many researchers believe this reason alone explains why the regular practice of slow, deep breathing has been shown to reduce your risk of heart disease, improve lung function, better oxygenate the blood, and improve your ability to exercise!

A slower breathing rate of six breaths a minute has also been shown to increase feelings of calmness and well-being. When you breathe rapidly and shallowly—using only the top of your chest— arteries throughout your body constrict. This reduces blood flow not only to the skin but also to the brain. This lack of blood flow triggers the stress response, making you feel tense and irritable. This can become a vicious cycle, as the resulting tension can cause you to breathe even more rapidly and shallowly.

Finally, slow and deep breathing helps you rid the body of acids, toxins, and carbon dioxide and flood the body with energizing oxygen. The more oxygen you bring into the body, the more energy every cell in your body can produce.

Try it and see for yourself. Put down the book and try to breathe as rapidly and shallowly as you can for a minute. How do you feel?

Tired? Anxious? Less focused? Now try it again. This time try to breathe slowly and deeply, bringing the air all the way into your lower belly and fully exhaling all of the breath. To breathe deeply and slowly, do the following:

1. Fully exhale, but without strain.

2. Fully and slowly inhale. As you inhale, bring the air down into your belly, feeling your navel and belly area rise upward with the breath.

3. Once your belly can no longer expand, bring the breath into the middle part of your lungs, by expanding your rib cage outward. You should feel the span of your ribs on your sides growing wider.

4. Bring the air into the top of the lungs, by allowing your breastbone and collarbones to rise upward.

5. Fully exhale.

6. Repeat five or six times over the course of one minute.

How do you feel? Focused? Joyful? I'm willing to bet that you have a lot more energy than you did five breaths ago! Indeed, breathing is more effective than napping!

Practice deep breathing once or twice a day. To remind yourself, set an alarm on your watch, or link your deep-breathing session with a natural break in your day. You might do it as you wait for your computer to boot up, as you wait for your coffee to drip into the pot each morning, or when you sit down in the train, bus, or cab for your morning commute. You might even schedule a couple of breathing breaks into your day, taking one midmorning and another midafternoon. Trust me, they'll be time well spent—you'll get more done because you'll be more productive and focused.

If in the beginning it feels painfully awkward to breathe slowly, just know that it will become more comfortable over time. You are building a skill, one that takes practice. It may help to try any or all of the deep breathing techniques that follow.

Three-part breathing. Don't worry about how quickly or slowly you are breathing. By bringing the breath into the lowest parts of your lungs, your breathing rate will naturally slow down. Lie on your back. Extend your legs, bend your knees, or elevate your feet and calves on a chair. Get your body as comfortable as possible.

Then place one hand on your lower belly, near your navel. Place the other hand on your chest, just above your breastbone. Breathe. Notice which hand moves. Does just the top hand move, or do they both move equally? This will give you some information about how you breathe.

Now let's work on deepening the breath. Take both hands and place them on your ribs. Breathe into your hands, expanding your rib cage outward as you breathe. You should actually feel a nice, soothing stretch along the middle of your back. Once you can no longer expand your rib cage, then bring the air into your chest and allow your breastbone to rise upward. Do this five or six times.

Now let's do a complete breath. Place one hand on your lower tummy, near your navel. Keep the other hand on one side of your rib cage for feedback. When you take your next breath, breathe into your lower hand, making your belly rise upward with the breath. Once you can lift your lower hand no farther, focus on the hand that's on your rib cage. Expand your rib cage outward. Once you can expand your ribs no more, move one hand to your chest and feel it rise as you fill your upper lungs with air. Then fully exhale and repeat as many times as needed. This should feel wonderful!

Breath counting. Some people feel uncomfortable when they first try to breathe deeply. This discomfort often stems from not fully exhaling, as it's uncomfortable trying to bring more oxygen into already full lungs. This exercise will help you to learn how to more fully exhale.

Sit comfortably. Bring your attention to your breath. Mentally count how long it takes you to inhale (one one hundred, two one hundred . . .) and how long it takes you to exhale. Do this two or three times. Then try to change your exhalations, making them last longer than your inhalations. You might make it your ultimate goal to exhale twice as long as you inhale. For today, go easy on yourself and just try to exhale one count longer than you inhale. So if you inhale for four counts, then exhale for five. If you inhale for five, exhale for six.

As you count, your breathing rate will probably naturally slow down, so don't focus too much energy on trying to breathe slowly. Instead, focus only on comfortably lengthening your exhalations. That will allow you to automatically lengthen your inhalations.

Mindful breathing. Sit comfortably and bring your awareness to your breathing. Don't do anything to change your breathing. Don't try to slow it down or to breathe more deeply. Rather, investigate and get to know the breath. Notice how it feels as it comes in and out of your nostrils. Notice what parts of your body expand and relax with the breath. What sensations do you notice as you inhale? What do you notice as you exhale? In particular, try to put your complete mental focus on the start of the inhalation, the end of the inhalation, the start of the exhalation, and the end of the exhalation.

By focusing on the breath but not consciously trying to change it, you will trigger your relaxation response. This, in turn, will automatically slow and deepen your breathing. As an added bonus, neuroscientist Candace Pert, Ph.D., believes that mindful breathing puts you in touch with the conversations going on between and among the cells in your body. You'll find that you are more in touch with your feelings, emotions, body tension, and desires, creating a type of intuition that will allow you to make better, more confident life decisions.

Recite the rosary or a mantra. Research completed at the University of Pavia in Italy has shown that recitation of the rosary prayer or the yoga mantra *"om mani padme om"* naturally slows the breath cycle down to six breaths a minute. By the way, study participants were normal, everyday folks who breathed quickly. Before reciting the rosary or chant, they were breathing fourteen times a minute. So whatever your religious persuasion or spiritual direction, if you enjoy prayer, meditation, or yoga chanting, give it a try.

LAUGHTER

STOP AGING PRESCRIPTION: AT LEAST ONCE A DAY

As we age, we lose our sense of humor. Babies begin to giggle by their fourth month of age, and some experts estimate that preschool-age young children laugh roughly four hundred times a day. Yet most adults laugh only seventeen or fewer times a day. This is despite the fact that many different studies have uncovered the powerful health benefits of laughter.

Studies show, for example, that a good belly laugh reduces levels of stress hormones in the body. It also boosts levels of neuropeptides that soothe away pain and boost mood. Laughter also bolsters immunity. It even exercises your heart and lungs, naturally squeezing stale air out of your lungs. Laughter cleanses your mind of negative emotions and stress and your body of stress hormones and the acids they produce.

For all of those reasons, regular doses of laughter help you to live longer. In a study of three hundred people completed at the University of Maryland Medical Center in Baltimore, people with heart disease were 40 percent less likely to laugh in a variety of situations compared to people of the same age without heart disease. Other studies have linked laughter with improved blood vessel health.

How do you go from someone who hardly laughs at all to someone who laughs contagiously? Try any of the following laughter-producing techniques.

Laugh with others. Laughing is infectious. Have you ever been in a lecture or another serious situation (a religious service, perhaps) when one person thinks of something a little bit funny but tries to avoid laughing? You see this person holding in the laughter and it makes you want to laugh. Quickly the entire room is laughing.

Laughter is social, so make it social. Consider designating a "laughter night" or a "funny time" during the day with your family or with a close friend. Be creative about how you get one another to laugh. You might play laughter-producing games, such as Twister. You might tickle one another. You might take turns telling your funniest joke or making your funniest face. You might sit around and reminisce about funny experiences you've had in the past. Or you might read the comics together or watch funny movies together.

Watch comedies rather than tragedies. Instead of revving up your stress response by watching crime shows and other serious dramas on television, gravitate toward sitcoms and other shows that make you laugh. You might keep on hand a DVD or video collection of the funniest movies of all times. Personally I love Mel Brooks, and I have all of his films in my collection. Not long ago I was listening to *The 2000 Year Old Man* in my car. It was the first time I had heard it in years and I cracked up. I was laughing so hysterically that people couldn't tell whether I was laughing or crying. I had tears streaming down my face.

CHILL OUT

STOP AGING PRESCRIPTION: TEN MINUTES, TWICE A DAY

In chapter 4 you learned how chronically elevated stress hormones can accelerate aging. To bring down stress hormones, you need to practice the art of turning on your relaxation response.

Regular doses of relaxation will teach you what it feels like to be relaxed. So many of us set off our stress response so often that we don't know what calm feels like. Once you know what calm feels like, you'll also more easily notice tension and other indications of stress and be able to halt your stress response more quickly.

Learning to relax will also help you dial into the internal communications going on inside your body all the time. We humans tend to be outwardly focused beings. Our minds stay occupied with work, family issues, and other aspects of life. Rarely if ever do we take the time to focus inward. Yet when we do bring our attention inward—say, to notice our breathing, our emotions, our bodily sensations—we cultivate a sixth sense, a type of bodily intuition. Learn to relax and you'll more easily integrate your whole body, optimizing your neuropeptide response and cell communication.

How do you relax? That's a great question. Relaxation can be elusive. For some people, it involves a formal practice or yoga, deep breathing, or meditation. I don't really care how you do it. Just spend some time every day by yourself. Sit and listen to soothing music or a meditation tape. Consider trying the following relaxation techniques.

Window gazing. Sit somewhere in a comfortable position where you can see out a window. Take five slow, deep breaths to relax. Then focus your attention on sights outside the window. Beauty surrounds us all the time, but we often don't notice it. See if you can notice—without labeling or using mental words to describe it—all of the natural beauty out the window. How do the leaves reflect light or move in the breeze? What wildlife do you see? How do different-colored pieces fit together?

Body scan. Lie on your back. Take a few slow, deep breaths. Then bring your awareness to your scalp, noticing any sensations. Slowly expand your awareness to your face, forehead, and skull.

How do your eyes feel? How do your cheeks feel? Do not try to physically relax any body area; just notice how it feels.

Slowly bring your awareness down your body, into your neck, your chest, then your right shoulder, right arm, right wrist, right hand. Continue until you've explored your entire body from head to toes.

Progressive muscle relaxation. This technique is similar to the body scan, except instead of simply noticing bodily sensations, you will actively try to relax your muscles. It's usually easiest to start at your feet and move upward to your head. As you inhale, tense up your feet as much as you can, squeezing your toes together. Then as you exhale, release the tension. Do the same with your calves, inhaling as you tense them up, and exhaling as you release. Move up to your thighs, then your abdomen, your sides and back, your chest, your shoulders and upper back, your arms, your hands, your neck, and your face.

GIVE BACK

STOP AGING PRESCRIPTION: AS OFTEN AS POSSIBLE

One of the best ways to bolster your joyful neuropeptide response is to help someone in need. We humans feel great after we've done a good deed. Many studies show that altruistic behaviors—giving blood, donating time to charity, teaching an adult to read—improve mental and physical health.

Don't make giving a "required" activity that adds stress to your life. That's not the point. Choose a way to give back to humanity and the earth in a way that makes you feel good. You might help to obedience-train or walk (or pet or bathe) dogs at the local animal shelter. You might help build or repair homes for people who are less fortunate.

You can give back in a formal way—by volunteering for a charity or organization—or you might give back in a much less formal way by doing a good deed every day. If you see a mother struggling to keep her toddler under control in the checkout line at the grocery store, you might help her unload her cart. If you see an elderly person with a cane struggling to walk down some steps, you might offer a hand to steady him or her. If you see someone struggling to change a tire, you might offer to help or call someone who can.

Make Yourself a Priority

Now that you've learned about the lifestyle prescriptions, I think it's time for a short pep talk. If you are like most of the patients who walk into my office, you're probably pretty good at meeting everyone else's needs but your own. You keep your boss happy by taking work home. You put aside your need for rest or quiet time to help your kids with homework and school projects. You stay up late listening to a friend's problems.

You probably know that your needs are important. You've probably heard that you can't effectively take care of others unless you first take care of you. You may even wholeheartedly believe it. Do you put the concept into practice?

When it comes down to it, most of us feel downright *guilty* taking time for ourselves. It's even a struggle for me sometimes. Yet carving out some "you" time to rest and restore is essential for lifelong good health and beautiful skin. It will take some effort to work these lifestyle prescriptions into your life. At first you'll find many seemingly good excuses for not finding the time. Persevere. Put aside your guilt and promise yourself some "you" time for fun, exercise, breathing, laughter, and relaxation. Doctor's orders.

8

the stop aging
skin care prescription

Your skin is the only outfit you wear every day, and it takes a beating. Regular doses of sunlight, air pollution, dry heating and air-conditioning, humidity, makeup, and hot showers regularly strip your skin of moisture, damage skin cell DNA, and interfere with important skin enzymes. Your Stop Aging Skin Care Prescription both protects the skin from future damage and reverses damage inflicted in the past by nourishing skin from the outside in.

Skin care products can quite effectively reduce wrinkles, brighten skin, even skin tone, reduce breakouts, and soothe away dryness and irritation. The problem is that there are too many products to choose from! You could easily get lost among the shelves and shelves of products at skin care superstores such as Douglas Cosmetics and Sephora. Even at discount stores such as Wal-Mart and pharmacies including CVS, it's easy to feel overwhelmed.

To help you make smarter, more confident skin care choices, I've created an insider's guide to the skin care aisle. In this chapter, you'll learn about the youth-promoting benefits of a number of skin care ingredients—including retinol, polyhydroxy acids (PHAs), vitamin E, vitamin C, soy, and copper, among many others. You'll learn, based on your age, skin type, skin color, and skin care needs, which of the latest ingredient technologies will help and which will not.

ASK DR. GRAF

Q: Are expensive skin care products more effective than discount products? I don't mind spending more money, but I want to know I'm getting what I pay for.

A: You need not go into debt in an attempt to look great. You can find most of the skin care products I recommend at discount stores such as Wal-Mart. In the vast majority of cases, the less expensive skin care products perform just as well as their $100 counterparts.

Let's start with the products you will need to use every day, up to twice a day.

Your Daily Routine

Research has shown that every part of your body, including the cells in your skin, follows a predictable pattern or daily cycle. During the day, skin cells perform different functions than they do at night. For this reason, your morning skin care routine should differ from your nighttime routine. Let's start with what you should do upon waking.

THE MORNING PRESCRIPTION

During the day, skin cells go into protection mode. In order to shield itself from the damaging effects of sunlight, your skin produces more sebum, with production peaking at noon. This oily substance delivers the antioxidant vitamin E to the skin's surface, helping to neutralize the damaging effects of sunlight and air pollution. The pH of the skin's surface is also higher during the day, allowing the skin to better protect itself from bacteria. For these reasons, your morning skin care routine emphasizes *protection*.

Each morning, follow these steps.

STEP 1:

Cleanse

To remove metabolic by-products produced by your skin cells overnight, wash your face in lukewarm water. Use your fingertips and not a Buf-Puf or other type of harsh scrub. Your fingers do a wonderful job of cleaning your skin, whereas scrubs can strip and irritate the skin. Use scrubs on your pots and pans, but not your face.

Do not shop for your cleanser in the deodorant soap aisle of the grocery store. That's where you'll find Dial, Irish Spring, and other soap bars, body washes, or deodorizing cleansers. These cleansers are extremely damaging to your skin. They are the equivalent of washing your face with Clorox bleach. Even pure soaps such as Ivory have a detergent-like effect, leaving the skin dry and stiff. You want a cleanser to remove sebum, but these soaps and deodorizing cleansers also break down your skin's moisture-retaining lipids. Unlike the inside of your body, the outermost layer of your skin functions best at a slightly acidic pH of 5. Many soaps and deodorizing cleansers, however, have an alkaline pH as high as 9. When you wash with an alkaline cleanser, the cleanser leaves an alkaline residue on your skin, which lasts for several hours. This disrupts the

---

A S K   D R .   G R A F

Q: I've been using a detergent soap to wash my face. I've tried more gentle, pH-balanced cleansers, as you recommend, but I never feel as if they are getting all the dirt and scum off my face. Do they really clean the face adequately?

A: Yes, they do. The problem lies in your definition of "clean." When you use a detergent cleanser, you are overcleaning the skin. In addition to dirt, makeup, and metabolic by-products, you are also scrubbing off your skin's naturally protective lipids. Your skin should not feel *dry* and flaky or red and raw after washing. It should feel soft and moist. All you need to effectively clean off dirt, excess sebum, scum, and makeup is the gentlest of cleansers and your fingertips. You do not need to scrub and scrub!

skin's naturally protective lipid barrier, causing moisture to quickly evaporate. During the several hours that it takes for the skin to repair its lipid barrier and return to its optimal pH, the skin is more vulnerable to outside influences.

Shop for your cleanser in the skin care aisle. You have your choice of foaming cleansers (which, in turn, come as lotions, creams, and gels), nonfoaming cleansers (which come in the form of creams, milks, and cold creams), and cleansing cloths. On top of that, some cleansers advertise active "youth-promoting" or "acne-reducing" ingredients such as alpha-hydroxy acids (AHAs), polyhydroxy acids (PHAs), and salicylic acids.

What type should you choose? Narrow down your choices by ignoring any product that does not list the words "pH balanced" somewhere on its packaging. This means that the product's pH is between 4 and 5.5.

Of the pH-balanced cleansers, pinpoint the best product for you based on your skin type. Use this guide:

• Normal and combination skin. Use a foaming cleanser designed for normal or combination skin.

• Oily and/or acne-prone skin. Look for a foaming cleanser that contains AHAs (such as lactic acid), salicylic acid, or (my personal favorite), polyhydroxy acids (PHAs). These ingredients will help to more easily break down and wash away excess sebum without causing irritation. They will also gently exfoliate your skin, leaving it fresh and radiant.

• Dry skin. Look for nonfoaming, oil-based "milky" cleansers designed specifically for dry skin. These cleansers are very gentle, more emollient, and hydrate as they clean.

• Darker skin. To avoid discoloration, you need a mild cleanser with a pH of at least 4. Investigate your cleanser's pH by calling the manufacturer's toll-free number listed on the packaging.

• Dry, sensitive, rash-prone skin. Look for a non-foaming cleanser with a slightly acidic or neutral pH that contains "nonionic surfactants." The packaging should advertise that the cleanser is designed for people with sensitive skin. Avoid cleansers that contain glycolic acid, particularly if the product has a pH below 4.0, as this ingredient can irritate your skin.

STOP AGING FACT

Oily skin tends to age more slowly than dry skin. The excess sebum that your sebaceous glands produce carries more vitamin E to the skin's surface. This helps to protect your skin from damage caused by sunlight and air pollution.

Change your cleanser with the changing seasons. If your skin is dry in the winter but normal or oily in the summer, you'll need different cleansers for different seasons. Notice how your skin changes and change your cleanser accordingly.

STEP 2:

Moisturize and Protect

You might wonder why step 2 jumps right to moisturizing. Shouldn't you use a toner first? Not necessarily. Today, facial cleansers are already pH-balanced, so using a toner is no longer necessary. When toners are applied, the "dirt" that you see on the cotton swab is not dirt at all. It is the top layer of dead skin cells. Removing them with a toner can strip moisture-retaining lipids further and cause irritation and discoloration.

Moisturizer is another story. It doesn't matter whether your skin is dry, oily, combination, or normal. You need moisturizer to replace moisture lost during cleansing and seal in that moisture so it does not escape. Your skin type may affect what *type* of moisturizer you use, but not whether or not you use it.

Moisturizers replace lost water and hold it there with humectants (water-binding agents). In other words, they add moisture to your skin and prevent existing moisture from escaping. Although your skin naturally retains moisture through small molecular weight compounds called natural moisturizing factor (NMF), it needs a layer of fatty acids (lipids) above the NMF layer to seal in this moisture and prevent it from evaporating. Showering, cleansing, sun exposure, wind, dry heating and air-conditioning, swimming, and other factors remove these fatty acids on a nearly constant basis. If you don't use a moisturizer to replace this lipid layer and seal in NMF, your skin's natural moisture evaporates, resulting in dry, thin, tight, older-looking skin.

Moisturizer is important for everyone of every age, but it becomes more important the older you get. The moister your skin, the smoother its texture and appearance. The smoother its texture, the better your skin reflects light. The better your skin reflects light, the more radiant you look. A good moisturizer not only hydrates the skin but also plumps it up, smoothing the appearance of fine lines.

Look for a moisturizer that advertises an SPF of at least 30. During the winter months, when UVB rays are weakest, you can get away with an SPF of 15. This SPF will protect your skin from sun damage during short outdoor activities, such as going to and from the car. Apply it first thing in the morning rather than waiting until you are ready to head outdoors. Although glass blocks sunburn-inducing UVB rays, it does not block much of UVA. Your SPF protection will last about an hour, so reapply (or touch up your mineral makeup, which also provides some sun protection) before going outdoors later in the day.

Make sure the sunscreen and/or sunblock in your moisturizer is broad-spectrum, with wording on the packaging that says it protects against both UVB and UVA rays. UVB rays are the ones that cause sunburn and skin cancer. UVA rays cause wrinkling, skin aging, and also contribute to cancer. As an added bonus, any antioxidants in your moisturizer (vitamins C, E, grape seed extract, or green tea) will enhance the protection from your sunblock as well as provide protection from environmental pollutants.

Finding the perfect moisturizer may take some trial and error. Try store samples whenever possible, and trust your instincts. If your skin feels shiny or greasy, the moisturizer is too rich for your skin type. If your skin feels tight and dry, it's not rich enough. If you have combination skin, you may need two different moisturizers—a gel or sheer sunscreen for the oily areas and a thicker moisturizer for the drier areas. If you have very dry skin, you may need to double your efforts, both using a rich moisturizer that contains no SPF or anti-wrinkle ingredients and applying a separate SPF product on top. This first layer moisturizer should contain humectants and emollient lipids such as ceramides and evening primrose oil. Evening primrose oil is the richest source of gamma-linolenic acid, a type of essential fatty acid that is soothing and particularly moisturizing for the skin.

STEP 3:
Protect Your Eyes

The skin around the eyes contains no oil-producing glands, making it thinner, more fragile, and more easily wrinkled and irritated than the skin on the rest of the face. Do not apply your facial moisturizer to the skin around your eyes. These moisturizers contain water, which the skin around your eyes will absorb, creating a puffy appearance.

Instead, use an eye cream on the eye area. These creams are richer than facial moisturizers and are made with ingredients that are safer and less irritating for this delicate skin. Choose an eye cream depending on what cosmetic concerns you wish to address:

• For crow's feet and crepiness, use a cream that contains collagen-producing peptides.
• If you have dark, puffy circles, use a cream that contains soothing natural ingredients such as soy, cucumber, or arnica.
• For dryness and general aging, use a cream that contains PHAs, retinol, and/or antioxidants.

Of course, if you are like me, you'll apply two or three different eye creams to treat multiple pet peeves, either layering them on or rotating them. Apply a pca-sized amount around the eyes in smooth, gentle strokes.

STEP 4:
Stand-Alone Sunscreen/Sunblock (for Extended Outdoor Time)

The SPF in your moisturizer along with any natural SPF in your makeup (see Step 5) will get you to and from your car and up and down the street for short stints outdoors. If you will be outdoors for an extended period of time, apply a stand-alone product that contains sunscreen and sunblock, as these technologies work differently. Sunblock ingredients (titanium dioxide and zinc oxide) generally block light from reaching the skin's surface. Chemical sunscreens generally absorb and denature sunlight, preventing it from causing damage. If you have sensitive skin, however, some sunscreens may irritate your skin, so you may need to opt for physical sunblock-only products instead.

Apply sunscreen/sunblock twenty minutes before heading outdoors, and reapply non-water-resistant versions every hour and water-resistant versions every ninety minutes.

Choose a product that:

• Is formulated for faces. These products will not clog your pores or trigger acne breakouts.
• Blocks UVA light. UVA light penetrates deeply into the skin and is the major contributor to skin damage, wrinkles, freckling, age spots, and skin discoloration. This type of sunlight is just as prevalent in the winter months as it is in the summer. It can also penetrate clouds and reflect off other surfaces to reach your skin, even if you are in the shade. If the product blocks UVA, it will contain one or more of the following ingredients: zinc oxide, titanium dioxide, or avobenzone. Note that zinc oxide and titanium dioxide may leave a bluish cast if you have darker skin. Instead, look for products that contain avobenzone, a UVA block. This ingredient needs photostabilization to prevent it from degrading in sunlight. Good products with this technology are made by the L'Oreal and Aveeno brands and are listed in the appendix.
• Has a high SPF. The SPF of a product is an indication of its ability to block UVB rays. When you will be spending a lot of time in direct sunlight (the beach, skiing on the slopes, gardening outdoors during the summer), use an SPF of 45 or higher. In the winter at sea level, you can get away with a lower SPF of about 15.
• Contains antioxidants. Antioxidants such as vitamins C and E, green tea polyphenols, and grape seed extract work with sunscreen to enhance sun protection. Unlike sunscreen, they also can protect your skin from damage caused by environmental pollutants. Look for a sunscreen that contains multiple antioxidants rather than just one, as they act synergistically.

When you are outdoors, follow these additional sun protection pointers:

• Wear sunscreen all year round, not just during the summer. UVA rays are just as damaging during the winter as they are during the summer.

• Wear sunscreen even if you'll be in the shade or it's cloudy.

• Reapply your sunscreen/sunblock after sweating or swimming, even if the product says it's waterproof. Make reapplication easier and less cumbersome by using a broad-spectrum UVA/UVB high-SPF spray, which requires no rubbing.

• Take cover. No sunscreen or sunblock is 100 percent protective. Some sunlight will still get through, despite your best efforts. So, whenever possible, shield yourself from direct sunlight. When walking or exercising outdoors, wear a hat with a visor. When on the beach, sit under an umbrella. When at your child's soccer game, cheer from the shade of the nearest tree.

STOP AGING TIP

Have you ever taken a winter vacation to Florida or the Caribbean only to burn or tan despite fanatical use of sunscreen/sunblock? It's not unusual for many people to burn during their first major sun exposure of the season, despite obsessively applying sunscreen/sunblock. I call it the "virgin effect." Over time, sunscreen/sunblock accumulates on your skin. Just one day of application provides some protection, but that protection is not always adequate for a first major sun exposure after you have been hibernating for several seasons. Multiple days of application provide more protection. I suggest that you apply sunscreen/sunblock all over your face and body for at least one week and ideally one month before a sunny vacation or your first summer sun exposure. This will allow the product to build up on your skin, providing you with maximum sun protection.

STEP 5:

Makeup (Optional)

If you wear makeup, I strongly suggest you give mineral makeup a try. Available online and in stores under different brands (consult the appendix for a list of my favorites), mineral makeup is made from colored minerals (mica, titanium dioxide, zinc and iron oxides) and ultramarine pigments that exist in nature. Because of the high mineral content, this type of makeup naturally kills bacteria. Even without preservatives, it maintains a long shelf life. It's preservative-free and has natural anti-inflammatory effects, making it perfect for people with sensitive or acne-prone skin.

The minerals in the makeup also reflect sunlight like a mirror, giving the makeup a natural SPF factor of about 15 to 20. For this reason, it's a great idea to touch up your makeup before heading outdoors. For mature skin, mineral makeup is sheer and covers well. Unlike other types of makeup, it does not clump up and accentuate existing wrinkles.

In addition to using mineral makeup whenever possible, try these additional makeup tips.

• Do not use waterproof mascara. It's difficult to remove, even with eye makeup remover, and can irritate your eyes, causing redness and puffiness. If your eyes are very sensitive, use only mineral makeup eye shades, which are much less irritating than regular eye makeup.

• Avoid creamy foundations if you have oily, acne-prone skin. They are heavy and can clog your pores.

• If your makeup is not mineral makeup, replace it every three months. Change your mascara more frequently.

• Never share makeup, especially mascara, with friends.

• Clean your brushes regularly.

STOP AGING TIP

If your skin care products have changed in color or texture, they are oxidizing and it's time to throw them away.

THE EVENING PRESCRIPTION

As you sleep, your body turns down or turns off many processes (digestion, most brain activity, etc.) so it can turn up the repair and renewal process. This renewal process takes place throughout your body, affecting every organ, including your skin. This is one reason why sleep is so important to good health.

At night, blood flow and lymphatic drainage increase, carrying more nutrients and energy to skin cells and hauling away more metabolic waste. The skin's pH also drops, which signals enzymes that repair and renew the skin to become more active.

Because of this, your nighttime skin care routine is designed to support this natural renewal process by providing the skin with the nutrients, moisture, and hydration it needs.

STEP 1:

Cleanse

Anyone who has ever lived with me or shared a hotel room with me knows that I am fanatical about washing my face at night. I've been this way ever since the day my older sister was married. I was eighteen, and, for some reason I kept excitedly running to the bridal room that night to reapply my mascara. By the end of the evening, I looked as if I had tarantula legs coming out of my eyes! I got home really late, and collapsed into bed without removing my makeup. One of my friends called me at 1:00 P.M. the next day. When my mom woke me to get me to take the call, I couldn't open my eyes. The mascara had dried and clumped together, gluing my eyelids shut! Ever since that day, I've kept moisturizing wipes by my bedside table. On those really late nights when I just want to fall into bed, I swab my face with a wipe. I'll skip my other skin care steps periodically, but cleansing is a must.

Cleansing is even more critical at night than it is in the morning. You might not be able to see and feel it all, but dust, germs, pollutants, dead skin cells, oil, and metabolic by-products have all collected on your skin throughout the day. You need to remove all of this, as well as any makeup and the residue of skin care products (moisturizer, sunscreen) that you applied in the morning. Otherwise your night products won't be able to fully penetrate the skin.

Think of what happens to dirty dishes when they sit in the sink overnight. What you could have easily washed off with minimal scrubbing later hardens into a caked-on substance that takes lots of elbow grease to remove. The same is true of your skin. Without nightly cleansing, I doubt you'll fully remove dead skin cells and sebum. Some of it will remain, disrupting skin pH and metabolism, leading to clogged pores, acne, and dullness. Your skin will be more vulnerable to injury, too.

Use the same cleanser at night as you do in the morning. If you wear makeup, you may need more cleanser and you may need to use slightly more finger action to thoroughly remove your makeup. Yet you can and should be gentle with your skin. Don't overwash—it can damage your skin or strip it of its natural oils.

STEP 2:

Moisturize and Renew

Use a different moisturizer at night than you use in the morning. At night, your skin is renewing itself, so you need a moisturizer that helps the skin to perform this important function. That comes down to one important ingredient: retinol. This highly studied skin care ingredient has been proven to even skin tone, promote elasticity, build collagen, and renew skin cells, promoting the birth of new skin cells as well as protecting the ones that already exist. It's the most important skin care ingredient, apart from sunblock, no matter your age, complexion, or skin type.

Retinol is a natural form of the vitamin A that is found in yellow and green vegetables, egg yolks, and fish oils. It's the most abundant form of vitamin A found in the skin. We learned about the benefits of retinol in the 1970s, when researchers began using it to treat acne. They noticed a side benefit to people who used Retin-A (a very strong prescription form of retinol). Their skin began to look younger. Retin-A seemed to reverse sun-induced aging in the following ways:

- Decreasing fine lines and wrinkles
- Improving collagen production
- Enhancing elasticity
- Improving skin tone and texture
- Enhancing skin lightening and minimizing age spots

It was most effective on the people who needed the most help— on skin that already had suffered lots of premature aging due to sun exposure. Retin-A is not available over the counter. You need a prescription for it. Over-the-counter retinol moisturizers, however, have also been shown to reduce wrinkles and other signs of aging— and without all of the irritating side effects of prescription Retin-A.

To choose a retinol moisturizer, follow these tips:

• To avoid redness or irritation, start with the lowest retinol cream you can find, slowly working your way up to increasingly stronger creams.

• Look for a retinol cream that is formulated for sensitive skin.

• Buy a cream from a respected cosmetic company to ensure stability and safety. Respected companies include Johnson & Johnson, Neutrogena, and Roc. Consult the appendix for a complete list of quality retinol creams.

• Don't stop using retinol once your appearance improves. You need to keep using retinol to maintain the results.

STEP 3:

Renew with Additional Beauty Products (Optional)

Retinol is one of the most important skin-renewing ingredients you can use. If you are a no-fuss type of person and know you won't be able to find the time to apply more than one product at night, then stick to retinol. Apply it and go to bed. On the other hand, if you are the type of person (like me) who will do everything you can to improve your appearance, then look for additional nighttime skin care products that address your most important skin care needs.

Wrinkle-Reducing Ingredients

Copper. It stimulates the production of collagen to decrease wrinkles, sagging, and roughness.

Peptides. Matrixyl (pentapeptide) helps to stimulate collagen production. In one study, a cream that contained Matrixyl decreased skin roughness by 27 percent, wrinkle volume by 36 percent, wrinkle depth by 50 percent, and wrinkle density by 68 percent over four months. Look for a cream that contains between 4 and 8 percent Matrixyl for maximum effect.

Another peptide called Argirelene (acetyl hexapeptide-3) may relax muscles in the face that lead to expression wrinkles (furrowing of the brow, for example). Some people have even touted it as the non-needle form of Botox. I wouldn't go quite that far, but this active ingredient does show promise.

Ingredients That Reduce Dullness, Blotchiness, Age Spots, and Uneven Skin Tone

AHAs and PHAs. When alpha-hydroxy acids (lactic acid, glycolic acid, citric acid, malic acid) first hit the market, everyone was wild about them. They were the first skin care products that really made a difference, so they quickly created high consumer demand. Soon, just about all skin care products—cleansers, moisturizers, peels, you name it—contained AHAs. They were in *everything*. As my patients began using more AHAs, however, their skin actually began to look chalky and dull. As it turned out, glycolic acid, the AHA ingredient that was most effective at exfoliating, tended to come packaged in a low-pH product. The chronic use of these low-pH products as well as excessive exfoliating in general activated collagen-degrading enzymes, which led to the chalkiness.

In working with patients over time, I've determined that there are some people who should never use AHAs. For everyone else, once-weekly use is about all the skin can handle. For daily exfoliation, PHAs are the much better choice, especially if you're over forty. PHAs (gluconolactone and lactobionic acid) provide all of the benefits of AHAs but are much gentler on your skin. PHAs smooth skin texture, cause dead skin cells to flake off, lighten the skin, even skin tone, and add and retain skin moisture. Look for a PHA in a serum rather than a cream, as it will penetrate the skin more effectively.

Soy. Unpasteurized soy milk has been shown to lighten uneven patches in the skin, reducing the appearance of age spots and other discolorations. It can also help to balance combination skin. Although soy is found in many products, practically all of them are made with fermented soy. The fermentation or pasteurization process destroys enzymes, making these products less effective. Only nonfermented soy (available solely in the Aveeno and Roc brands) contains the enzymes needed to lighten skin pigmentation and discolorations.

STEP 4:
Eye Cream

Reapply your eye cream at night, using the same one you used in the morning.

STOP AGING TIP

If your retinol product once worked beautifully but now irritates your skin, throw it away. Retinol is very sensitive to light and air. When it oxidizes, it becomes irritating and harmful.

Weekly and Monthly Prescriptions

Each day when you wash your face, you gently remove dead skin cells, revealing the softer, more radiant skin beneath. Periodically you need to follow up with more intensive exfoliation to more completely but gently strip skin of dead cells.

Why do you need to exfoliate? When you were a child, enzymes in your skin functioned at their peak, naturally triggering dead skin cells to flake off. This is why young children look so radiant and why their skin glows. Their skin exfoliates naturally.

As you age, however, the skin loses its natural moisture, which prevents exfoliating enzymes from working as effectively. Dead skin cells remain stuck rather than flaking off, preventing the skin from reflecting light. End result: your skin looks dull, ashy, and gray.

As you age, you need to give your exfoliating enzymes a helping hand. At the same time, you don't want to get overly aggressive. Scrubbing your skin or using overly strong exfoliating methods will not only remove the top layer of dead cells but also strip the skin of *all* of the layers of dead cells and even some live cells. Without these protective skin cell layers, your skin cannot seal in its moisture, so it becomes drier. This irritates your skin, causing exfoliating enzymes to work even less effectively than before.

How to Exfoliate

Exfoliate as often as once a week or as infrequently as once a month, depending on your age and skin texture. If you are younger than age forty and have oilier, more hydrated skin, your exfoliating enzymes may still be doing an adequate job of sloughing off dead skin cells. They may not build up quickly, so once-monthly exfoliation may be all you need. On the other hand, if you are older than forty and have drier skin, your exfoliating enzymes may barely be active at all, so you may need to exfoliate as often as weekly. Use this rule of thumb: if your skin starts to look dull or ashy, it's probably time to exfoliate. On the other hand, if your skin starts to look red and irritated, you're either exfoliating too much or using overly harsh methods.

You can exfoliate at home, or you can do it at a spa by getting a facial, peel, or microdermabrasion. Just stick to one exfoliating method. Don't double up with a microdermabrasion and a peel. That's too much. Do one or the other and stick with the same method over time.

Just as you would do a bit of research before lining up a hair stylist, look into the aesthetician before you make an appointment. Your aesthetician should be licensed in your state. You should know people who glowingly recommend her or him, and whoever you choose should have been in the business for many years.

EXFOLIATION METHODS

To exfoliate, use one of the following methods. Start by exfoliating once a month, slowly progressing to as often as once a week. Follow package directions, never using more than the instructions recommend. Always start with the gentlest dose or shortest time and progress from there. If your skin is red and irritated after a treatment, the exfoliating method was too harsh. Your skin should never look worse before it looks better. Ideally, you should look in the mirror after exfoliating and love what you see! You should not be embarrassed to be seen in public.

You have a choice between two basic types of exfoliation: chemical peels and microdermabrasion.

AT-HOME OR IN-OFFICE CHEMICAL PEELS

Chemical peels lift off dead skin cells. There are many types of peels, and the best type for you may vary by skin type and complexion. At-home peels are generally weaker than peels you would get at a spa. Spa peels are weaker than peels used at a dermatologist's office.

Here's a rundown on the different types.

Alpha-hydroxy acid peels (usually glycolic acid peels). These particles are very small, so they penetrate the skin rapidly, which can cause irritation, skin discoloration, and redness in some people. Use extra care with chemical peels if you have darker skin, dry skin, or sensitive skin.

There are various types of AHA peels, ranging from the gentlest lactic acid and glycolic acid to the strongest phenol (available only at a dermatologist's office). The pH of an at-home AHA peel should be higher than 3.5 to avoid irritation. The pH won't be listed on the product, so call the manufacturer's toll-free number listed on the product packaging and ask. If the customer service representative on the other end of the line doesn't know the pH, ask him or her to find out. I can't stress this enough. Don't use a product until you know for sure.

Enzyme peels. Made from the enzymes found in papaya (papain) and pineapple (bromelain), these peels work better for people with sensitive skin. Newer enzyme technologies such as Actizyme are now becoming available thanks to improved shelf life.

MICRODERMABRASION

Microdermabrasion is a procedure where a small vacuuming device is combined with the exfoliating action of tiny, perfectly spherical crystals. A number of new at-home kits, when used properly, are quite effective at buffing and polishing the skin. The spherical smooth quality of the aluminum oxide crystals used in microderm-abrasion kits will not injure the skin or break skin capillaries (as do the sharp edges found in scrubs).

Special Advice for Adult Acne

Yes, despite popular belief, acne does not just torment teenagers with raging hormones. I've even treated postmenopausal women with acne.

Although adult acne stems from causes similar to those that provoke teen acne, you need very different products to treat it. As an adult, you no longer have the oily skin of most teens. Your skin cannot tolerate the harsh, drying acne products that line the skin care shelves of many drugstores and supermarkets. Not only can these products create itchy, flaky, red skin, they can actually lead to more acne. I believe in skin comfort. I do not believe that your skin must get worse before it gets better. You do not have to go through an ugly, icky stage where you look like you've been kissed by a porcupine before your acne finally clears up.

Look for products designed specifically for adults that contain no or very little (no more than 2.5 percent) benzoyl peroxide. This ingredient can dry adult skin, especially in products that include higher percentages. Also, higher amounts of this ingredient can dry, irritate, and bleach darker skin tones.

Daily cleanser. Use a daily cleanser that contains alpha-hydroxy acids to prevent clogged pores. If you have sensitive or darker skin, use one with gentler polyhydroxy acids or salicylic acid.

Breakout cleanser. When you have a breakout, switch to a gentle cleanser that contains salicylic acids. This will help clear up a breakout more quickly. These cleansers should be no stronger than a 2 percent solution. Once you've cleared up the breakout, switch back to your usual cleanser.

Breakout moisturizer. Use Aveeno Clear Complexion moisturizer, which contains a blend of salicylic acid and a nonfermented soy product. These ingredients will reduce the redness and inflammation of a pimple.

Cleansing wipes. Use astringent pads such as the brand Stridex to cleanse your face—especially the T-zone area—during and after exercise, when traveling on a hot train, or in other situations that cause excess oil production.

In addition to those products, get in the practice of using ice to shorten the duration of a pimple. At the first sign of a blind pimple (a pimple you can feel but can't yet see), apply ice. This will constrict the blood vessels in the area of the pimple, reducing inflammation. This can shrink the size of the cyst and shorten its course.

Below-the-Neck Care

For reasons I've already stated, you *need* to cleanse your face twice a day. Your body, on the other hand, remains under cover most of the day and night. Unlike your face, the skin on your body is not constantly exposed to dirt, smog, and airborne particles. You also have no makeup or beauty products to remove. Less sebum production also keeps it from getting as greasy. So, unlike your face, you do not need to wash your body as often. Ideally, you should minimize your body skin's exposure to water as much as possible.

To understand why, imagine living in a place where it rained torrentially for fifteen to twenty minutes every day, 365 days a year. Picture what the outside of your house would look like after just one year, especially if you had neglected to paint or seal the wood, replace the shingles on the roof, or caulk the windows and doorways. Eventually the paint would fade and chip, your roof would leak, and wind would seep through your windows and doors. Now think of how it would look ten, twenty, or thirty years later.

Daily showering ages your skin just as daily rain ages the outside of a house. Showering strips your skin of its protective lipid layer, allowing moisture to evaporate. This results in dryness, itchiness, and irritation. It also creates dry, brittle nails. Take no more than one shower a day, and consider cutting back to just once every other day. If you plan to exercise on any given day, shower after exercising, not first thing in the morning.

Keep your shower as short as possible, just three to five minutes. To ensure you get out of the shower on time, purchase either an egg timer or a shower radio to time your bathing; if using a radio, hold your shower to one song. Consider staying under the stream of water only long enough to wet down your body and rinse. Step out of the stream or turn off the water to lather your body and hair and to shave.

In addition to cutting back on shower time, also stay away from other sources of water. Never use a hot tub. If you like to relax in one after a gym workout, use the sauna or steam room instead.

If your skin does not feel silky smooth within two weeks on this plan, you may need to shower less often. Cut back to as few as two showers a week. You may be surprised to find that your body remains odor-free much longer than you may expect. If odor is an issue, use a washcloth or cleansing wipes to spot clean problem areas such as feet, armpits, and genitals. Just stand in the tub with the water running, clean those areas, and then step out of the tub. Also, check out the Deodorizing Powder recipe, page 206.

When showering, follow this advice:

• Shower with clean water. Put a filter on your showerhead. If you have hard water, consider putting in a water softener as well. Chlorine in tap water is an oxidative agent (that's how it kills bacteria) and may dry the skin.

• Use lukewarm water. Hot water removes natural skin oils more quickly and increases evaporation of moisture from skin by causing skin blood vessels to dilate.

• Use a nondrying, pH-balanced cleanser. Detergent-based cleansing bars and soap such as Dial, Safeguard, and Irish Spring are too alkaline and will dry your skin. If you feel you must use one of these products to control odor, use it only on odor-causing areas such as your underarms. Don't inflict damage on the rest of your skin.

Purchase your shower gel or bar in the beauty aisle (in the same place you find your moisturizer). You'll want a product that is labeled "non-soap cleanser." The label "moisturizing" should also appear on the packaging.

I personally love non-soap cleansers made from salt or sugar and oil. Available at many day spas and bath stores, the sugar in these cleansers gently exfoliates without stripping skin of its natural oil layer, and the oil seals in moisture. Plus these gentle salt and sugar scrubs smell fantastic, and, as I've mentioned before, if you smell good, you'll feel good, and if you feel good, you'll look good. You'll find some of my favorite make-at-home scrub recipes on pages 206–209.

STOP AGING TIP

If you have oily, acne-prone areas on your chest and back, swab these areas with a cleansing or astringent wipe after your shower. These wipes will remove excess sebum without overly stripping the skin.

Now, I would be remiss if I didn't anticipate that some of you will be reluctant to give up your favorite soap. You may like the way you smell afterward or how the soap foams up. Non-soap cleansers universally do not foam up the way soap-based cleansers do. This addiction to foam is something you need to break. Trust me. You are getting just as clean without the foam. Dry skin is not the same thing as clean skin. When you get out of the shower, you want to feel moist, not dry.

Every Morning and Evening

To moisten your skin below the neck, apply moisturizer twice a day. If you take a shower daily, apply moisturizer right after showering, as this will seal in any water that remains on your skin. You'll moisturize in two steps.

Layer 1. Use a lotion that contains urea or lactic acid. Apply it liberally from neck to toe. These ingredients are found in the skin's NMF and act as humectants to attract moisture into the skin.

Layer 2. Massage body oil or a thicker lotion over the first layer. Use a natural oil such as almond oil, avocado oil, coconut oil, shea butter, hemp oil, or CeraVe (a ceramide cream). These penetrate the

---

ASK DR. GRAF

Q: I swim for fitness. What can I do to combat the drying effects of my favorite form of activity?

A: In addition to immersing yourself in water, you are also exposing your skin to chlorine, which is very drying. To keep your skin moist, shower quickly right after getting out of the pool to remove any chlorine residue. If you swim daily, make this the only shower you take that day. On the days that you don't swim, skip the shower.

When you shower, use a non-soap, moisturizing cleanser such as Cetaphil. After showering, gently pat your skin dry, allowing it to remain moist. Immediately apply your two layers of moisturizer. Be vigilant and liberal with moisturizer. You may need as many as three applications daily to keep your skin moist.

skin better than synthetic oils made from petroleum (such as baby oil). Natural oils seep into your skin, creating a silky-smooth texture rather than leaving you feeling greasy. Plus they emulate the skin's natural lipid barrier, locking in moisture. To moisturize your body in a hurry, use a natural oil body spray. It's faster to apply, and you can more easily get it on your back and other hard-to-reach areas.

Outdoor Body Care

Sunlight ages the skin on your body just as it ages the skin on your face. Use a broad-spectrum sunblock that protects against UVA and UVB rays. It should have an SPF of at least 15 in the winter and 45 in the summer. If it contains any antioxidants such as vitamins C and E, green tea polyphenols, or grape seed extract, consider it a bonus.

Apply it generously all over your skin. Whenever in doubt, use more, as studies consistently show that people underapply sunscreen. Slather it on twenty minutes before going outdoors and reapply every hour. When you reapply—especially if you are on the beach or exercising and sweating a lot—do yourself a favor and use a sunscreen spray that does not have to be rubbed in. Reapply after swimming or sweating a lot, too, even if you're using a water-resistant variety.

Stay in the shade as much as possible and wear a hat to shield your face.

Softer, Smoother Hands

Your hands come into contact with water more times a day than you probably realize. This continually strips them of their moisture, leaving hands dry, cracked, itchy, and sore. I'm not suggesting you live an unhygienic lifestyle, but you can take one very effective step to limit how often you expose your hands to water. In two words: surgical gloves. Buy yourself a box of powder-free latex or vinyl surgical gloves. If I can use them to perform detailed surgical techniques, you can use them to cook, chop vegetables, and clean the house. As an added bonus, they will protect the skin on your hands from irritants that are often found in garlic, onions, and hot peppers, not to mention the irritants in household soaps and cleaning products. When the gloves become dirty, wash the outsides of the gloves while you are wearing them, just as you would normally wash your hands.

In addition to protecting your hands from water, you also want to seal in moisture. Purchase a number of hand creams. They are labeled as such and are thicker and richer than body or facial moisturizers. Place hand cream in strategic places (at every sink, in your handbag or briefcase, at your desk, in the car) and use it as often as possible.

Finally, we've all been told to wash our hands religiously to avoid passing germs. Use hand sanitizer instead of soap and water whenever possible. It kills viruses and other germs just as effectively, without overly drying your hands.

LESS BRITTLE NAILS

The same tactics that keep the skin on your hands soft and moist will also protect your nails. Avoid water and apply moisturizer often. Also take care when giving yourself a home manicure or getting one at a salon. Try the following suggestions:

• Use polish sparingly. Go ahead and paint your nails for special occasions, but allow them to go natural the rest of the time. Nail polish prevents moisture from evaporating from your nails. When the moisture gets trapped, yeast and fungal infections more easily take hold. Also, putting on polish means that you eventually need to take it off with polish remover, which is irritating and drying to the nails. Irritation can cause them to split, peel, and become brittle.

• Don't overly shape your nails. Cut them straight across, rounding them slightly at the tip. If you file them into points, you will weaken them, causing them to break more easily.

• Don't cut your cuticles. The cuticle forms a seal between the nail and the skin, preventing irritants from gaining access. If you clip, remove, or push back the cuticle, you set the stage for bacterial or fungal infection. Instead, use a cuticle cream, especially in the winter months, to prevent them from becoming dry, brittle, or cracked.

• If you get manicures at a salon, bring your own tools or store them at the salon. Manicure and pedicure tools and implements that have not been properly sterilized can spread viral infections such as HIV, hepatitis B and C, and warts.

Your Best Face

I hope, after reading this chapter, you feel more confident about purchasing skin care products. For specific product advice, consult the appendix. Keep in mind that your skin care routine will evolve over time. As you change your diet and lifestyle and balance your body pH, your skin will change, too. Dry skin may become moister. Oily skin may become normal. Dull skin will brighten. As a result, you may need different skin care products three months from now than you need today. You also will probably find that you'll need to update your skin care products each season. During the dry winter months, you'll need to use a heavier moisturizer than during the humid summer months. Whenever you look in the mirror and say to yourself, "Hmmm, I just don't look great," it's time to reassess your products. It's time for a change.

9

two weeks to a younger you

The Stop Aging, Start Living Plan works *instantly*. I'm not kidding. I've seen the dramatic and instantaneous results in patient after patient after patient. Quite often, when someone walks into my office and looks haggard and dull, I mix an Alkalinizing Cocktail and serve it on the spot. By the end of the appointment, my once dull and tired patient has already transformed into a vibrant, brighter, more energetic person.

You don't need to travel to my office in New York to experience this transformation. You need only commit yourself to following the four prescriptions outlined in this book. It doesn't matter what genetics you inherited from your parents, even if every woman in your genetic lineage sprouted frown lines, crow's feet, and age spots before her thirtieth birthday. It doesn't matter if you did everything wrong until this very moment—sunbathing with baby oil slathered all over your body, smoking, following a meat-and-potato-chips diet, somehow living on two hours of sleep each night, or setting off your fight-or-flight response fifteen times every minute. It doesn't matter if you repeatedly did all of those things for years. You can stop aging—right now.

You can erase up to five years overnight. That's right. This program is so effective that you will see a change in your appearance by tomorrow morning.

Grow Younger Overnight

Depending on how quickly you want to see results and on how motivated you are to make dietary and lifestyle changes, you will implement the Stop Aging plan in one of three ways.

If you want to see fast, dramatic results: Start the Stop Aging plan fast with the 24-Hour Kick-Start (page 136). It requires quite a bit of planning, effort, and tenacity, but the tough part lasts only twenty-four hours. More important, you'll feel and look unbelievably fantastic in the morning, erasing up to five years.

If you want reasonably fast results, but don't want to do anything uncomfortable to get them: Start on Day 1 of the 2-Week Plan (page 147). On this slower-paced plan, you will still see results, but they won't be as immediately dramatic.

If the idea of making many lifestyle changes at once triggers your stress response: See my Baby Steps plan, (page 171). It will help you to prioritize the Stop Aging Prescriptions from most important to least, so you can focus on making just one or two changes at once.

A Word About Withdrawal Symptoms

No matter which of the three plans you use, your body will undergo a gentle detoxification process, cleansing itself of excess acids that have built up and been stored in fat tissue under the skin. Depending on how much acid has been building up in your body, your initial detoxification process may create a few temporary side effects. Usually these side effects last just a few days. Many people don't notice them at all. The severity of your side effects, along with their duration, will depend on the severity of the acid and toxin buildup in your body. The healthier you are when you start the program, the fewer symptoms you will have. The sicker you are, the more pronounced the withdrawal will be.

You may experience any of the following temporary symptoms:

Fever
Headache

Muscle and joint discomfort, especially first thing in the morning

Pasty mouth

Trouble concentrating

Fatigue

Skin rashes and acne

Mood swings

The following optional strategies will reduce the severity of withdrawal symptoms as well as help to improve the detoxification process.

Start the program during an "easy" week. It's probably not ideal to start the plan while you are moving to a new home, changing jobs or careers, starting a family, going through a divorce, or otherwise under a lot of chronic, ongoing stress. Start the plan when you have some time to devote to yourself. Most important, you need to be able to rest. The first two weeks of the plan are the most critical. The rest will ensure that your body has the energy it needs to focus on neutralizing and eliminating stressors. The quiet time will give you the mental space that you need to absorb new lifestyle habits.

Drink a Cleansing Cocktail (page 205) daily. You only need the Cleansing Cocktail during weeks 1 and 2 of the program. To make it you'll need a good juicer, which is a wise investment in your health. It contains apples, carrots, kale, beets, and ginger to speed detoxification.

Take a liver tonic. Sold in health food stores under various brands, liver tonic supplements help to support liver detoxification. They generally contain any or all of the following ingredients: milk thistle, any number of powdered cruciferous vegetables (broccoli, Brussels sprouts, cauliflower), dandelion, taurine, psyllium, and slippery elm bark. Good brands include Liver Care (from Himalaya Herbal Healthcare) and A-F Betafood, by Standard Process, Inc. Check with your doctor before taking this or any other supplement, especially if you are being treated for a medical condition or taking prescription medications.

Double up on Alkalinizing Cocktails. After the first two weeks on the program, you'll maintain your results with just one Alkalinizing Cocktail a day. During the first two weeks, however, you may need an extra cocktail, especially if you notice withdrawal symptoms. To improve the cocktail's detoxification power, consider adding extra spirulina or chlorophyll (both sold in health food stores) to the drink.

Relax in a sea salt bath once a day. Normally I do not promote sitting in a tub full of warm water because it can dry the skin. Yet sitting in a warm bath is wonderfully relaxing and soothing. During week 1, the benefits of relaxation far outweigh the risks of drying your skin. Just take smart countermeasures by using a good body moisturizer after the bath.

When you add sea salts to the bath, you turn your bath into an alkalinizing spa experience. Sea salts will draw acids out of the body through the skin. To make the salt bath, fill the tub with warm water. Add 2 cups of baking soda (which contains alkalinizing bicarbonate) and 2 cups of sea salt. (Epsom salts will also work in a pinch.) Soak for twenty to thirty minutes. Drain the water, rinse off quickly in the shower, pat dry, and apply body lotion and oil.

Sit in a sauna or steam room. The dry heat of the sauna or moist heat of the steam room will induce sweating, allowing you to release toxins through the skin. Set the heat in the sauna high enough to induce sweating but not so high that you can't stand to stay inside for forty-five minutes. Shower afterwards to wash released toxins off your skin. Do not use a sauna if you are obese, are pregnant, have hepatitis, or are anemic.

Sign up for a body wrap. Many spas offer sea salt scrubs and herbal body wraps. These wonderfully relaxing treatments help to pull toxins out of the body through the skin.

Sign up for a massage. Massage stimulates the flow of lymph through the body. You might think of lymph as the sanitation workers of the human body. When you stimulate lymph flow, garbage (germs, toxins, wastes) gets picked up and transported out of the body more quickly. Massage also involves skin-to-skin contact, and touch is very healing and comforting. The warmth and energy of someone's hands against your skin can be particularly healing during the initial weeks of detoxification.

My most important word of advice for weeks 1 and 2 of the rest of your life? *Persevere*. If you continue to follow the program, you will soon feel amazing. Feeling good is contagious. Once you experience the jolt of energy from your alkalinizing lifestyle, you'll never want to go back to your old way of living.

The 24-Hour Kick-Start

Okay, you've decided to accelerate your results by following the 24-Hour Kick-Start. During the next twenty-four hours, you will eat *only* alkalinizing foods, you'll practice a number of alkalinizing and stress-reducing lifestyle habits, and you'll take a few cleansing supplements to more quickly detoxify your body.

I'm not going to sugarcoat this. The 24-Hour Kick-Start is challenging. Although it does not require fasting, it does require that you eat no meat, no sugar, and no grains for twenty-four hours. You'll also have no alcohol, cola, or coffee. Instead, you'll consume fruits, vegetables, avocado, nuts and seeds, fruit and vegetable juices, and lemon water. You also will follow your various Stop Aging Prescriptions to a T. You'll take all of your recommended Stop Aging supplements and complete all of your recommended Stop Aging lifestyle activities and Stop Aging skin care routines. You'll also use additional supplements and self-pampering activities to further speed your results.

I recommend you do the Kick-Start on a day off from work. If you are a parent, try to get a sitter, family member, or friend to watch your children for most of the day. You might even sign the kids up for a weekend-long camp. Clear your calendar of all to-do items. Make this a day that you focus only on what's good for you. Don't spend the day doing laundry, washing dishes, or catching up on other chores. Your Kick-Start isn't a chore. It's a gift.

I also recommend you keep your landline, pager, and cell phone turned off most of the day. Use your phone to call out, if needed, but don't keep it on to allow others to call in. Let's face facts. If the phone rings, you'll be tempted to pick it up. If you pick it up, someone invariably will talk you into doing something—and there goes your gift.

I also recommend you avoid doing anything stress-producing. Don't watch the news. Don't read the paper (except for the comics and other enjoyable sections). Stay away from e-mail. Try to stay out of your car and out of traffic. If possible, try not to deal with people who annoy you.

Spend the day doing all of the things that you love but never find time to do. Read the novel that has been sitting unopened on your nightstand. Call that friend who always makes you laugh. Dig in your garden (but only if you enjoy it—not because the weeds annoy you). Take a nap. Sit outside and listen to the sounds of birds chirping. Put on your favorite music. Do something really fun. Have you decided on your fun activity yet? I hope so! Treat yourself to something extravagant. Get a massage, a seaweed wrap, or some other luxurious but detoxifying spa treatment. It will help induce your relaxation response (perhaps even generate some joyous neuropeptides) as well as speed the removal of toxins from your body.

Below you will find a detailed description of your 24-Hour Kick-Start. If you have a health condition such as diabetes, please check with your health care provider before taking the supplements recommended in the Kick-Start. If you have a blood glucose disorder, choose only low-glycemic-index fruit (berries, melon, apples, and pears) for between-meals snacks.

7:00 A.M. (UPON WAKING)
❑ Morning skin care prescription
    • Cleanser
    • Moisturizer
    • Eye cream
    • Sunblock
❑ Body care: moisturizer all over your body, topped with body oil
❑ Test your saliva pH
❑ 5 minutes of deep breathing
❑ Probiotic supplement
❑ Alkalinizing Cocktail
❑ 2 spirulina capsules, 500 milligrams each
❑ Liver tonic supplement
❑ 16 ounces filtered water with lemon or lime

7:30 A.M. (BREAKFAST)
❑ Unlimited amount of fresh fruit
❑ Cleansing Cocktail

8:00 A.M. (AFTER BREAKFAST)
❑ Mineral supplement with calcium
❑ 16 ounces filtered water with lemon or lime
❑ 20–30 minute walk outdoors pushing the pace comfortably

10:00 A.M. (SNACK)
❑ Unlimited amount of fresh fruit

11:00 A.M. (SNACK)
❑ Any recipe from the juicing section of chapter 10 or a freshly squeezed store-bought juice

NOON (LUNCH)
❑ 1 huge salad made with dark leafy greens, assorted veggies of your choice, ⅓ cup almonds and seeds (pumpkin seeds are wonderfully alkalinizing), and Alkalinizing Salad Dressing (see page 200)
❑ Huge side of any alkalinizing cooked vegetable of your choice (sautéed greens, steamed broccoli, cooked cauliflower, Brussels sprouts)

1:00 P.M. (AFTER LUNCH)
❑ mineral supplement with calcium
❑ Relax for 10+ minutes

3:00 P.M. (SNACK)
❑ Unlimited amount of any raw vegetables
❑ 2 spirulina capsules, 500 milligrams each
❑ 16 ounces filtered water with lemon or lime

3:30 P.M.
❑ 5 minutes of deep breathing

4:30 P.M.
❑ Alkalinizing Cocktail

6:00 P.M. (DINNER)

❑ 1 huge salad made with dark leafy greens, unlimited assorted veggies of your choice, $\frac{1}{2}$ medium avocado, sliced, and Alkalinizing Salad Dressing (page 200)

❑ Huge side of any alkalinizing cooked vegetable of your choice (sautéed greens, steamed broccoli, cooked cauliflower or Brussels sprouts).

6:30 P.M. (AFTER DINNER)

❑ Relax for 10+ minutes

6:45 P.M. (SNACK)

❑ Unlimited amount of fruit

❑ 2 spirulina capsules, 500 milligrams each

❑ 16 ounces filtered water with lemon or lime

7:00 P.M.

❑ Watch a funny movie or sitcom or go to a comedy club—do something guaranteed to produce laughter

9:00 P.M.

❑ Sea salt soak: Spend 20–30 minutes soaking in a tub filled with 2 cups baking soda, 2 cups sea salt, and lukewarm water

❑ Night skin care prescription

• Cleanser

• Retinol serum

• Eye cream

• Any additional optional age-reducing creams (collagen-producing peptide cream, soy cream, vitamin C cream, etc.)

❑ Test your saliva pH

9:30 P.M. TO 7:00 A.M.

❑ Sleep

7:00 A.M. (NEXT DAY)

❑ Look in the mirror

❑ Test your saliva pH

❑ Start the Stop Aging program on day 1 (page 147)

Your 2-Week Plan

Did you try the 24-Hour Kick-Start? If so, how do you look and feel? Do you notice a new brightness to your eyes, glow to your skin, and radiance to your complexion? Are you amazed at how much better you can look and feel in just one day? The changes you saw in the first twenty-four hours are only a taste of the results to come. From here, it only gets better.

If you did not try the Kick-Start, you're about to prove something to yourself. By tomorrow morning you will know without a doubt that it really doesn't matter how much junk you've eaten over the course of your life, how little you've paid attention to your skin, or how stressful your lifestyle has become. As soon as you take charge of your beauty and health, your cells respond—instantly. Your organs, tissues, and cells want to work with you. They want to be in an alkaline state. Give your cells the ingredients they need to function optimally and that's exactly what they will do.

During each of the next fourteen days, you will improve the way your cells communicate with one another. You'll cleanse your cellular fluids of acids and other barriers to cell communications and energy production, and you'll create the optimal environment for skin cells to work at their peak. As a result, you'll create more vibrant, more youthful skin.

Although the plan certainly takes commitment and dedication, I can promise you that you won't be living like a monk and forcing yourself to eat twigs. Not only do I prescribe this plan to my patients, I also live it. I drink coffee, enjoy a glass of wine with dinner, don't always eat enough fruit or vegetables, and live a very stressful life full of teenagers, travel, and work commitments. This plan allows for these indiscretions. Although I challenge you to try to follow it 100 percent for at least the first two weeks, you'll still see amazing results if your best is just 80 percent. The plan is that powerful. It's not only very effective; it's also simple, achievable, and affordable.

Get Ready

Before starting the plan, make sure you have on hand everything you need for success. I've created this convenient shopping list for you.

SUPPLEMENTS

Benefiber or Fiber-sure

Mineral supplement with calcium

Greens powder

Optional: Organic lemonade or apple juice

Optional: Spirulina

Probiotic supplement

EQUIPMENT AND SUPPLIES

Egg timer or shower radio (to time your showers)

Juicer

pH test strips

Water filter for your sink (drinking water) and showerhead

SKIN CARE PRODUCTS

Body cleanser

Body lotion

Body oil

Eye cream

Facial cleanser

Facial moisturizer for morning

Facial sunblock

Hand cream

Optional: Additional youth-promoting facial skin care products, such as soy creams, vitamin C creams, collagen-producing peptide creams, etc.

Retinol serum for night

FOOD

Keep the following ingredients on hand at all times. This is by no means an exhaustive list, but it will ensure you have most of what you need. You'll only need to shop for the fresh ingredients used in various recipes.

IN THE PANTRY

Apple cider vinegar

Assortment of raw nuts and seeds (almonds, cashews, pecans, macadamia nuts, sunflower seeds, pumpkin seeds)

Balsamic vinegar

Bananas

Canned chickpeas and white beans

Coconut flakes

Extra-virgin olive oil

Flaxseed meal

Garlic

Lentils

Oatmeal

Onions

Peanut oil

Peppercorns

Pure maple syrup

Quinoa

Raisins

Sea salt

Sesame oil

Spices: cinnamon, curry, etc.

Vegetable and chicken stocks

Wild rice

Whole-grain bread (best choice: bread made with oat flour)

Whole-grain pancake mix

Whole-grain pasta (see appendix)*

Whole-grain, high-fiber cereal (see appendix)**

* Brands: Annie's Homegrown Whole Wheat, Barilla Plus, Heartland Multigrain or Whole Grain, Hodgson Mill Whole Wheat, Mueller's Multigrain

** Brands: Kellogg's All Bran, General Mills Fiber One, Kashi GoLean (e.g., Good Friends), Post 100% Bran Cereal, Nature's Path Organic Flax Plus Multibran

IN THE REFRIGERATOR

Assortment of organic fresh vegetables (bell pepper, carrots, celery, Brussels sprouts, broccoli, etc.)

Assortment of organic fruit (apples, pears, mango, etc.)
Assortment of organic greens (kale, cabbage, dark lettuce varieties, bok choy, etc.)
Lemons and limes
Lowfat milk or almond milk
Organic eggs

IN THE FREEZER
Assortment of frozen vegetables

GET SET

Do the following either the night before or the morning you start the plan:

1. Place a pH test strip (consult the appendix for recommended brands) on your tongue and record the results.

2. Take a "before" photo and then store it away. You'll compare this photo to another that you take in two weeks. Wear no makeup for the photo. Also, make a note of your outfit, time of day, and the location where the photo is taken. In two weeks, you'll want to take your "after" photo in the same lighting, location, and outfit for an accurate comparison.

3. Take the "Test Your Aging Potential" self-assessment on page 144. You will fill out this assessment again in two weeks.

IMPLEMENT THE 2-WEEK PLAN

For each of the next fourteen days, you'll find detailed lifestyle checklists to help you make your Stop Aging Supplement, Lifestyle, and Skin care Prescriptions a habit. Each day appears like a day planner, with tasks filled in according to the time of day. Keep in mind that the time to complete each task is just a suggestion. Use each day's activities as a guide in helping you to fill in your own appointment book or to-do list. Feel free to move activities to different times during the day, or even to different days.

Test Your Aging Potential

Take the following true-or-false quiz before you start the program. I recommend you photocopy the quiz rather than write in the book, as you will be using this again. Mark a T next to each statement that resonates with you and an F next to each one that doesn't.

_ *I get moody.*
_ *My face gets blotchy.*
_ *I toss and turn at night.*
_ *I break out easily.*
_ *My skin looks dull.*
_ *My skin feels dry.*
_ *I suffer from allergic skin rashes.*
_ *I look older than my age.*
_ *I feel older than my age.*
_ *I am prone to constipation and gas.*
_ *I feel cold most of the time; I wear sweaters when everyone else is in short sleeves.*
_ *My joints feel achy when I wake in the morning.*
_ *I have periods of mental fog when I can't concentrate.*
_ *I feel under pressure to do things.*
_ *I feel tense at work.*
_ *I am filled with a sense of dread.*
_ *Something is missing in my life.*
_ *I hate getting out of bed in the morning.*

On this quiz, "false" answers are your ultimate goal. Don't fret if you answered "true" to most or all of the questions. I guarantee that when you retake this quiz in just two weeks, you'll answer "false" to many more. As you stay on the program for life, periodically retake this quiz to help stay on track. If you notice your results are slipping (you answered "true" to a question that you had answered "false" to earlier), see it as an opportunity to reexamine your eating, lifestyle, and skin care routine.

I've made each day's suggestions very specific. I don't just remind you to breathe; I suggest a specific breathing exercise. I don't tell you to laugh; I suggest how to make it happen. I've done this to encourage you to try new things. That said, if you already are in the habit of relaxing, meditating, or deep breathing, continue to do what works for you. The lifestyle recommendations in this 2-Week Plan are just that—*recommendations*. Feel free to change the suggested exercise, breathing, and other lifestyle activities to ones that suit you.

New York city nutrition expert Leslie Dantchik, M.S., designed each day's menu, ensuring that the options you find on each day not only are alkalinizing but also contain the ingredients to promote good digestion and brain health. Because it's an optional part of the plan, I have not separated fruit from suggested meals. If you find that your digestion improves when you consume fruit alone, then modify the menus accordingly. On any menu day, you may add any of the following snacks: fresh fruit, trail mix (raisins, sunflower seeds, pumpkin seeds, almonds, cashews, dried fruit of your choice), or raw vegetables (plain or dipped in guacamole). You may also include frozen grapes (page 202), or warmed sliced apples (page 203) as a dessert on any day of the plan. Choose other desserts in chapter 10 only one to two times a week.

As with the lifestyle recommendations, use these menus as a rough guide, not as a dietary edict. Use them to get a detailed understanding of three-to-one eating and not to torture yourself into the tedium of following unfamiliar recipes day in and day out. You do not need to follow these menus in order. Go ahead and mix and match the breakfast, lunch, and dinner options. If you're like me, you might even eat the same option many days in a row.

Keep in mind that these menus reflect a balance of acid-producing and alkalinizing foods. To help you stay in balance, I've included serving sizes for acid producers such as coffee, meat, and sugar-containing foods. Eat as many alkalinizing vegetables, greens, and fruit as you desire.

I'll see you in two weeks. Good luck, and remember: if you stray from the plan, enjoy your splurge. Savor every bite and then recommit yourself. Don't set off your stress response by feeling guilty about it!

Easy Meal Makeovers

To make your own alkalinizing meals, use the following meal makeovers as a guide.

Breakfast

Instead of: Scrambled eggs with bacon
Have: Vegetable omelet, preceded by a side of fruit

Instead of: Low-fiber breakfast cereal and milk
Have: High-fiber breakfast cereal (see page 142) with almond milk, preceded by a piece of fruit

Instead of: Muffin, doughnut, or other pastry with coffee
Have: Alkalinizing muffin (see page 177) with freshly brewed espresso

Lunch

Instead of: Ham and cheese sandwich
Have: Open-faced ham and cheese melt on high-fiber bread and a huge salad preceded by a side of fruit

Instead of: Chicken wrap with side of chips
Have: Grilled chicken over salad and a side of baked sweet potato fries

Instead of: Tuna fish sandwich with fries or chips
Have: Tuna salad mixed with chopped veggies of your choice, served open-faced on toasted whole-grain bread with a slice of cheese; eat with a side salad

Dinner

Instead of: Steak with white rice
Have: Steak and vegetable stir-fry with wild rice

Instead of: French dip and fries
Have: Beef and vegetable stew with steamed broccoli

Instead of: BBQ chicken with corn bread
Have: 1 piece of BBQ chicken with any sautéed green and a
   salad

Dessert
Instead of: Any sugar-packed dessert
Have: Unsweetened applesauce with cinnamon, fresh fruit
   with homemade whipped cream (no sugar added), fruit
   dipped in dark chocolate, or any of the dessert recipes in
   chapter 10

DAY 1

7:00 A.M. (UPON WAKING)
❑ Morning skin care prescription
   • Cleanser
   • Moisturizer
   • Eye cream
   • Sunblock
❑ Body care: Moisturizer all over your body, topped with body oil
❑ Test your saliva pH
❑ Three-part breathing for 5 minutes
❑ Probiotic supplement
❑ Alkalinizing Cocktail
❑ 16 ounces filtered water with lemon or lime

7:30 A.M.
Breakfast: Omelet with Kale, Feta, and Yellow Tomato (page
             179)
             Sliced melon
             Freshly squeezed juice
             1 to 2 cups organic coffee or tea

8:00 A.M. (AFTER BREAKFAST)
❑ Mineral supplement with calcium
❑ 16 ounces filtered water with lemon or lime

NOON

Lunch: Potato Leek Soup (page 187) with whole-grain roll
Mixed Green Salad (page 196)

1:00 P.M. (AFTER LUNCH)

☐ Mineral supplement with calcium

3:00 P.M.

☐ 16 ounces filtered water with lemon or lime

6:00 P.M.

Dinner: Tricolor Green Salad with Tuscan-Style Strip Steak
(page 191)
Roasted Brussels Sprouts (page 197)

6:45 P.M.

☐ 16 ounces filtered water with lemon or lime

7:00 P.M.

☐ Relax in a sea salt soak: spend 20–30 minutes soaking in a tub
filled with 2 cups baking soda, 2 cups sea salt, and lukewarm
water; do 5 minutes of three-part breathing while you are in
the tub

☐ Watch a funny movie

9:00 P.M.

☐ Night skin care prescription
• Cleanser
• Retinol serum
• Eye cream
• Any additional optional age-reducing creams (collagen-
producing peptide cream, soy cream, vitamin C cream, etc.)

10:00 P.M. TO 7:00 A.M.

☐ Sleep

DAY 2

7:00 A.M. (UPON WAKING)

❑ Morning skin care prescription
- • Cleanser
- • Moisturizer
- • Eye cream
- • Sunblock

❑ Body care: moisturizer all over your body, topped with body oil
❑ Test your saliva pH
❑ Breath counting for 5 minutes
❑ Probiotic supplement
❑ Alkalinizing Cocktail
❑ 16 ounces filtered water with lemon or lime

7:30 A.M.

Breakfast: Greek-Style Yogurt with Grapes, Granola, and Blue-
              berries (page 181)
              Freshly squeezed juice
              1 to 2 cups organic coffee or tea

8:00 A.M. (AFTER BREAKFAST)

❑ Mineral supplement with calcium
❑ 16 ounces filtered water with lemon or lime

NOON

Lunch: Tuna with Jicama, Cilantro, and Lime (page 192)
          Apple

1:00 P.M. (AFTER LUNCH)

❑ Mineral supplement with calcium
❑ Body scan for 10 minutes

3:00 P.M.

❑ 16 ounces filtered water with lemon or lime

3:30 P.M.

❑ Breath counting for 5 minutes

5:00 P.M.
❏ Exercise of your choice

6:00 P.M.
Dinner: Whole-Grain Pasta with Greens (page 196)
              Mixed Green Salad (page 196)

6:45 P.M.
❏ 16 ounces filtered water with lemon or lime

7:00 P.M.
❏ Call friend who makes you laugh
❏ Relax in a sea salt soak

9:00 P.M.
❏ Night skin care prescription
    • Cleanser
    • Retinol serum
    • Eye cream
    • Any additional optional age-reducing creams (collagen-producing peptide cream, soy cream, vitamin C cream, etc.)

10:00 P.M. TO 7:00 A.M.
❏ Body scan for 10 minutes
❏ Sleep

DAY 3

7:00 A.M. (UPON WAKING)
❏ Morning skin care prescription
    • Cleanser
    • Moisturizer
    • Eye cream
    • Sunblock
❏ Body care: moisturizer all over your body, topped with body oil
❏ Test your saliva pH
❏ Mindful breathing for 5 minutes
❏ Probiotic supplement
❏ Alkalinizing Cocktail
❏ 16 ounces filtered water with lemon or lime

7:30 A.M.

Breakfast: ½ cup cottage cheese mixed with chopped melon, cinnamon, and sliced almonds

Freshly squeezed juice

1 to 2 cups organic coffee or tea

8:00 A.M.

❑ Walk outdoors up to 20 minutes

❑ Mineral supplement with calcium

❑ 16 ounces filtered water with lemon or lime

NOON

Lunch: Sliced grilled chicken (4 ounces) with fresh spinach, sliced mushrooms, 1 ounce goat cheese, and cranberries, tossed with olive oil and balsamic vinegar, sea salt and pepper

1:00 P.M. (AFTER LUNCH)

❑ Mineral supplement with calcium

❑ Sit quietly outdoors, listening intently to the sounds all around you, for 10 minutes

3:00 P.M.

❑ 16 ounces filtered water with lemon or lime

3:30 P.M.

❑ Mindful breathing for 5 minutes

6:00 P.M.

Dinner: Shrimp, Bok Choy, and Mixed Vegetables (page 195) over brown rice

Sliced pineapple

6:45 P.M.

❑ 16 ounces filtered water with lemon or lime

7:00 P.M.

❑ Relax in a sea salt soak

9:00 P.M.

❑ Night skin care prescription
  • Cleanser
  • Retinol serum
  • Eye cream
  • Any additional optional age-reducing creams (collagen-producing peptide cream, soy cream, vitamin C cream, etc.)

10:00 P.M. TO 7:00 A.M.

❑ Sleep

DAY 4

7:00 A.M. (UPON WAKING)

❑ Morning skin care prescription
  • Cleanser
  • Moisturizer
  • Eye cream
  • Sunblock
❑ Body care: moisturizer all over your body, topped with body oil
❑ Test your saliva pH
❑ Sing in the shower
❑ Probiotic supplement
❑ Alkalinizing Cocktail
❑ 16 ounces filtered water with lemon or lime

7:30 A.M.

Breakfast: Chai Tea Smoothie with Toasted Coconut and Banana
                   (page 178)
              Grapefruit
              Freshly squeezed juice
              1 to 2 cups organic coffee or tea

8:00 A.M. (AFTER BREAKFAST)

❑ Mineral supplement with calcium
❑ 16 ounces filtered water with lemon or lime
❑ Read the comics

NOON

Lunch: Sliced Turkey Crunch Sandwich (page 190)

              Asian Jicama Slaw (page 193)

              Orange

1:00 P.M. (AFTER LUNCH)

❑ Mineral supplement with calcium

❑ Window gazing for 10 minutes

3:00 P.M.

❑ 16 ounces filtered water with lemon or lime

3:30 P.M.

❑ Whistle while you work, up to 5 minutes

6:00 P.M.

Dinner: Seared Tuna (page 189) with sautéed escarole and

             Roasted Tomatoes (page 198)

7:00 P.M.

❑ Get out some instruments or the pots and pans and hold a family or personal jam session to your favorite music

❑ Relax in a sea salt soak

9:00 P.M.

❑ Night skin care prescription

   • Cleanser

   • Retinol serum

   • Eye cream

   • Any additional optional age-reducing creams (collagen-producing peptide cream, soy cream, vitamin C cream, etc.)

10:00 P.M. TO 7:00 A.M.

❑ Relax with a good book

❑ Sleep

DAY 5

7:00 A.M. (UPON WAKING)

❑ Morning skin care prescription
- • Cleanser
- • Moisturizer
- • Eye cream
- • Sunblock

❑ Body care: moisturizer all over your body, topped with body oil
❑ Test your saliva pH
❑ Three-part breathing for 5 minutes
❑ Probiotic supplement
❑ Alkalinizing Cocktail
❑ 16 ounces filtered water with lemon or lime

7:30 A.M.

Breakfast: Hard-boiled organic egg with an open-faced grilled
              cheese and tomato sandwich on whole-grain bread
              (use only 1 slice of cheese)
              Freshly squeezed juice
              1 to 2 cups organic coffee or tea

8:00 A.M. (AFTER BREAKFAST)

❑ Mineral supplement with calcium
❑ 16 ounces filtered water with lemon or lime

NOON

Lunch: Chopped Tofu Salad (page 183)
              Sliced cantaloupe

1:00 P.M. (AFTER LUNCH)

❑ Mineral supplement with calcium
❑ Listen to soothing music for 10+ minutes

3:00 P.M.

❑ 16 ounces filtered water with lemon or lime

3:30 P.M.

❑ Three-part breathing for 5 minutes

6:00 P.M.

Dinner: Turkey burger (4 to 5 ounces) with store-bought
              vegetable medley and Sweet Potato Chips (page
              198)

6:45 P.M.

❑ 16 ounces filtered water with lemon or lime

7:00 P.M.

❑ Dance to your favorite music 10+ minutes
❑ Relax in a sea salt soak

9:00 P.M.

❑ Night skin care prescription
   • Cleanser
   • Retinol serum
   • Eye cream
   • Any additional optional age-reducing creams (collagen-
   producing peptide cream, soy cream, vitamin C cream, etc.)

10:00 P.M. TO 7:00 A.M.

❑ Progressive muscle relaxation
❑ Sleep

DAY 6

7:00 A.M. (UPON WAKING)

❑ Morning skin care prescription
   • Cleanser
   • Moisturizer
   • Eye cream
   • Sunblock
❑ Body care: moisturizer all over your body, topped with body oil
❑ Test your saliva pH
❑ Probiotic supplement
❑ Alkalinizing Cocktail
❑ 16 ounces filtered water with lemon or lime

7:30 A.M.

Breakfast: Blueberry and Sunflower Seed Muffin with Flax (page 177)

                ½ cup nonfat or lowfat yogurt with raspberries (or your favorite berry)

                Freshly squeezed juice

                1 to 2 cups organic coffee or tea

8:00 A.M. (AFTER BREAKFAST)

❏ Mineral supplement with calcium

❏ 16 ounces filtered water with lemon or lime

NOON

Lunch: Avocado, Alfalfa Sprout, and Grilled Vegetable Sandwich (page 182)

           Grapes

1:00 P.M. (AFTER LUNCH)

❏ Mineral supplement with calcium

3:00 P.M.

❏ 16 ounces filtered water with lemon or lime

3:30 P.M.

❏ Breath counting for 5 minutes

5:00 P.M.

❏ Exercise of your choice

6:00 P.M.

❏ Breath counting for 5 minutes (before dinner)

Dinner: Beef Sirloin Stew with Parsnips (page 182)

           Mixed Green Salad (page 196)

6:45 P.M.

❏ 16 ounces filtered water with lemon or lime

7:00 P.M.

❏ Have a family joke night

9:00 P.M.

❑ Night skin care prescription

- Cleanser
- Retinol serum
- Eye cream
- Any additional optional age-reducing creams (collagen-producing peptide cream, soy cream, vitamin C cream, etc.)

10:00 P.M. TO 7:00 A.M.

❑ Sleep

DAY 7

7:00 A.M. (UPON WAKING)

❑ Morning skin care prescription

- Cleanser
- Moisturizer
- Eye cream
- Sunblock

❑ Body care: moisturizer all over your body, topped with body oil

❑ Test your saliva pH

❑ Probiotic supplement

❑ Alkalinizing Cocktail

❑ 16 ounces filtered water with lemon or lime

7:30 A.M.

Breakfast: Super Omega-3 Banana Pecan Pancakes with Honey
                     Butter and Maple Syrup (page 179)
                     Freshly squeezed juice
                     1 to 2 cups organic coffee or tea

8:00 A.M. (AFTER BREAKFAST)

❑ Mineral supplement with calcium

❑ 16 ounces filtered water with lemon or lime

NOON

❑ Mindful breathing for 5 minutes (before lunch)

Lunch: Curried Chicken Salad with Grapes and Macadamia
                 Nuts (page 184)

1:00 P.M. (AFTER LUNCH)

❑ Mineral supplement with calcium

❑ Find a funny joke on the Internet and e-mail it to a friend

3:00 P.M.

❑ 16 ounces filtered water with lemon or lime

3:30 P.M.

❑ Mindful breathing for 5 minutes

4:00 P.M.

❑ Reward yourself with a massage, seaweed wrap, pedicure, or other relaxing luxury

6:00 P.M.

Dinner: Broiled Scallops (page 183)

Wild rice (page 199 for basic cooking instructions) and steamed asparagus with lemon (page 177 for steaming instructions)

6:45 P.M.

❑ 16 ounces filtered water with lemon or lime

7:00 P.M.

❑ Sing silly songs ("If You're Happy and You Know It . . .")

8:00 P.M.

❑ Sea Salt Glow (page 209), followed by Peppermint and Lavender Foot Soak (page 208) and Revitalizing Foot Scrub (page 208)

9:00 P.M.

❑ Night skin care prescription

• Cleanser

• Retinol serum

• Eye cream

• Any additional optional age-reducing creams (collagen-producing peptide cream, soy cream, vitamin C cream, etc.)

10:00 P.M. TO 7:00 A.M.
❑ Sleep

DAY 8

7:00 A.M. (UPON WAKING)
❑ Morning skin care prescription
  • Cleanser
  • Moisturizer
  • Eye cream
  • Sunblock
❑ Body care: moisturizer all over your body, topped with body oil
❑ Test your saliva pH
❑ Three-part breathing for 5 minutes
❑ Probiotic supplement
❑ Alkalinizing Cocktail
❑ 16 ounces filtered water with lemon or lime

7:30 A.M.

Breakfast: Cooked oatmeal mixed with raisins, ground flaxseed,
            and sliced banana
            Freshly squeezed juice
            1 to 2 cups organic coffee or tea

8:00 A.M. (AFTER BREAKFAST)
❑ mineral supplement with calcium
❑ 16 ounces filtered water with lemon or lime

NOON

Lunch: Lunch at a Japanese restaurant (suggested meal: eda-
        mame, 1 or 2 sushi rolls, miso soup, and a salad
        with ginger dressing)

1:00 P.M. (AFTER LUNCH)
❑ Mineral supplement with calcium
❑ Window gazing for 10 minutes

3:00 P.M.
❑ 16 ounces filtered water with lemon or lime

6:00 P.M.

Dinner: White Bean and Chicken Chili (page 192) over couscous

6:45 P.M.

❑ 16 ounces filtered water with lemon or lime

7:00 P.M.

❑ Sea salt soak; spend 5 minutes of your soak practicing three-
part breathing

❑ Watch a funny movie

9:00 P.M.

❑ Night skin care prescription

- Cleanser
- Retinol serum
- Eye cream
- Any additional optional age-reducing creams (collagen-
producing peptide cream, soy cream, vitamin C cream, etc.)

10:00 P.M. TO 7:00 A.M.

❑ Sleep

DAY 9

7:00 A.M. (UPON WAKING)

❑ Morning skin care prescription

- Cleanser
- Moisturizer
- Eye cream
- Sunblock

❑ Body care: moisturizer all over your body, topped with body oil

❑ Test your saliva pH

❑ Breath counting for 5 minutes

❑ Probiotic supplement

❑ Alkalinizing Cocktail

❑ 16 ounces filtered water with lemon or lime

7:30 A.M.

Breakfast: 2 ounces sliced smoked salmon, sliced tomato, sliced
onion, and 1 tablespoon low-fat cream cheese on
1 slice of whole-grain bread

Mixed berries

Freshly squeezed juice

1 to 2 cups organic coffee or tea

8:00 A.M. (AFTER BREAKFAST)

❑ Mineral supplement with calcium

❑ 16 ounces filtered water with lemon or lime

❑ Walk outdoors for up to 20 minutes

NOON

Lunch: Sesame-Grilled Chicken Sandwich with Miso Mayonnaise and Cucumber Slaw (page 189)

Peach or nectarine

1:00 P.M. (AFTER LUNCH)

❑ Mineral supplement with calcium

3:00 P.M.

❑ 16 ounces filtered water with lemon or lime

3:30 P.M.

❑ Breath counting for 5 minutes

6:00 P.M.

Dinner: Sautéed Eggplant in Spicy Tomato Sauce (page 188)
over 1 cup whole-grain pasta

Mixed Green Salad (page 196)

6:45 P.M.

❑ 16 ounces filtered water with lemon or lime

7:00 P.M.

❑ Hold a contest to see who can make the funniest face

9:00 P.M.

❑ Night skin care prescription

- • Cleanser
- • Retinol serum
- • Eye cream
- • Any additional optional age-reducing creams (collagen-producing peptide cream, soy cream, vitamin C cream, etc.)

10:00 P.M. TO 7:00 A.M.

❑ Progressive muscle relaxation for 20 minutes
❑ Sleep

DAY 10

7:00 A.M. (UPON WAKING)

❑ Morning skin care prescription

- • Cleanser
- • Moisturizer
- • Eye cream
- • Sunblock

❑ Body care: moisturizer all over your body, topped with body oil
❑ Test your saliva pH
❑ Mindful breathing for 5 minutes
❑ Probiotic supplement
❑ Alkalinizing Cocktail
❑ 16 ounces filtered water with lemon or lime

7:30 A.M.

Breakfast: ¾–1 cup high-fiber cereal (page 142 for recommended brands) with skim or almond milk and 2 tablespoons dried dates or cranberries
Freshly squeezed juice
1 to 2 cups organic coffee or tea

8:00 A.M. (AFTER BREAKFAST)

❑ Mineral supplement with calcium
❑ 16 ounces filtered water with lemon or lime

NOON
Lunch: Lentil Soup (page 185)
            Mixed Green Salad (page 196)
            Pear

1:00 P.M. (AFTER LUNCH)
❑ Mineral supplement with calcium
❑ Body scan for 10 minutes

3:00 P.M.
❑ 16 ounces filtered water with lemon or lime

3:30 P.M.
❑ Mindful breathing for 5 minutes

6:00 P.M.
Dinner: Grilled wild salmon (flavor with Basic Fish Marinade,
               page 201)
            Steamed broccoli
            Pureed Butternut Squash (page 197)

6:45 P.M.
❑ 16 ounces filtered water with lemon or lime

7:00 P.M.
❑ Play Twister, Ring Around the Rosy, Red Light—Green Light,
   or any other active children's game with children or adults

9:00 P.M.
❑ Night skin care prescription
   • Cleanser
   • Retinol serum
   • Eye cream
   • Any additional optional age-reducing creams (collagen-
   producing peptide cream, soy cream, vitamin C cream, etc.)

10:00 P.M. TO 7:00 A.M.
❑ Read a good book
❑ Sleep

DAY 11

7:00 A.M. (UPON WAKING)
❑ Morning skin care prescription
  • Cleanser
  • Moisturizer
  • Eye cream
  • Sunblock
❑ Body care: moisturizer all over your body, topped with body oil
❑ Test your saliva pH
❑ Sing in the shower
❑ Probiotic supplement
❑ Alkalinizing Cocktail
❑ 16 ounces filtered water with lemon or lime

7:30 A.M.
Breakfast: Vanilla Mango Yogurt Smoothie (page 181)
              Scrambled organic egg with chopped chives
              Freshly squeezed juice
              1 to 2 cups organic coffee or tea

8:00 A.M. (AFTER BREAKFAST)
❑ Mineral supplement with calcium
❑ 16 ounces filtered water with lemon or lime

10:00 A.M.
❑ 10-minute walk

NOON
Lunch: Shrimp Garden Wrap (page 190)
              Quinoa Salad (page 199)

1:00 P.M. (AFTER LUNCH)
❑ Mineral supplement with calcium

3:00 P.M.

❑ 16 ounces filtered water with lemon or lime

❑ Whistle while you work

5:00 P.M.

❑ 10-minute walk

6:00 P.M.

Dinner: Pepper-Seared Yellowtail Tuna over Salad (page 187)
            Fresh cherries

6:45 P.M.

❑ 16 ounces filtered water with lemon or lime

7:00 P.M.

❑ Watch a sitcom

❑ Cuddle with a loved one

9:00 P.M.

❑ Night skin care prescription

   • Cleanser

   • Retinol serum

   • Eye cream

   • Any additional optional age-reducing creams (collagen-producing peptide cream, soy cream, vitamin C cream, etc.)

10:00 P.M. TO 7:00 A.M.

❑ Sleep

DAY 12

7 A.M. (UPON WAKING)

❑ Morning skin care prescription

   • Cleanser

   • Moisturizer

   • Eye cream

   • Sunblock

❑ Body care: moisturizer all over your body, topped with body oil

❑ Test your saliva pH

❑ Three-part breathing for 5 minutes
❑ Probiotic supplement
❑ Alkalinizing Cocktail
❑ 16 ounces filtered water with lemon or lime

7:30 A.M.
Breakfast: Toasted oat bran English muffin topped with 1 table-
                    spoon almond butter and sliced apple
                    Freshly squeezed juice
                    1 to 2 cups organic coffee or tea

8:00 A.M. (AFTER BREAKFAST)
❑ Mineral supplement with calcium
❑ 16 ounces filtered water with lemon or lime

NOON
Lunch: Mediterranean Crab Salad (page 186)
                    Sliced fresh tropical fruit (papaya, mango, pineapple)

1:00 P.M. (AFTER LUNCH)
❑ Mineral supplement with calcium
❑ Window gazing for 10 minutes

3:00 P.M.
❑ 16 ounces filtered water with lemon or lime

3:30 P.M.
❑ Three-part breathing for 5 minutes

6:00 P.M.
Dinner: Grilled chicken breast (see page 182 for basic cook-
                    ing instructions)
                    Braised Red Cabbage (page 194)
                    Baked sweet potato

6:45 P.M.
❑ 16 ounces filtered water with lemon or lime

7:00 P.M.

❏ Hold a "funny stories" night, reminiscing about the funniest occasions in your relationship with family and/or friends

9:00 P.M.

❏ Night skin care prescription
  • Cleanser
  • Retinol serum
  • Eye cream
  • Any additional optional age-reducing creams (collagen producing peptide cream, soy cream, vitamin C cream, etc.)

10:00 P.M. TO 7:00 A.M.

❏ Progressive muscle relaxation
❏ Sleep

DAY 13

7:00 A.M. (UPON WAKING)

❏ Morning skin care prescription
  • Cleanser
  • Moisturizer
  • Eye cream
  • Sunblock
❏ Body care: moisturizer all over your body, topped with body oil
❏ Test your saliva pH
❏ Breath counting for 5 minutes
❏ Probiotic supplement
❏ Alkalinizing Cocktail
❏ 16 ounces filtered water with lemon or lime

7:30 A.M.

Breakfast: Weekend brunch at restaurant or home (suggested meal: vegetable omelet, frittata, or organic poached eggs with 1 slice whole-grain bread and side of sliced melon)

1 to 2 cups organic coffee or tea

8:00 A.M. (AFTER BREAKFAST)
☐ Mineral supplement with calcium
☐ 16 ounces filtered water with lemon or lime
☐ Read the comics

NOON
Lunch: ¼ cup hummus over 2 cups field greens and mixed vegetables (sliced cucumber, cherry tomatoes, broccoli) with toasted whole-grain pita on the side

1:00 P.M. (AFTER LUNCH)
☐ Mineral supplement with calcium
☐ Breath counting for 5 minutes

3:00 P.M.
☐ 16 ounces filtered water with lemon or lime

3:30 P.M.
☐ Compliment a co-worker, friend, or family member, just to see them smile

6:00 P.M.
Dinner: 4 ounces broiled halibut
           Kale with Garlic and White Beans (page 196)
           Wild rice (page 199 for basic cooking instructions)

6:45 P.M.
☐ 16 ounces filtered water with lemon or lime

7:00 P.M.
☐ Dance to your favorite music

9:00 P.M.
☐ Night skin care prescription
  • Cleanser
  • Retinol serum
  • Eye cream

• Any additional optional age-reducing creams (collagen-producing peptide cream, soy cream, vitamin C cream, etc.)

10:00 P.M. TO 7:00 A.M.
❑ Body scan for 20 minutes
❑ Sleep

DAY 14

7:00 A.M. (UPON WAKING)
❑ Morning skin care prescription
  • Cleanser
  • Moisturizer
  • Eye cream
  • Sunblock
❑ Body care: moisturizer all over your body, topped with body oil
❑ Test your saliva pH
❑ Mindful breathing for 5 minutes
❑ Probiotic supplement
❑ Alkalinizing Cocktail
❑ 16 ounces filtered water with lemon or lime

7:30 A.M.
Breakfast: 2 whole-grain waffles (page 221 for recommended brands) topped with maple syrup and ½ cup sliced strawberries
Freshly squeezed juice
1 to 2 cups organic coffee or tea

8:00 A.M. (AFTER BREAKFAST)
❑ Mineral supplement with calcium
❑ 16 ounces filtered water with lemon or lime
❑ Go sightseeing on foot or bike

NOON
Lunch: Citrus Salmon Salad (page 184)
Whole-grain roll

1:00 P.M. (AFTER LUNCH)
❑ Mineral supplement with calcium

3:00 P.M.
❑ 16 ounces filtered water with lemon or lime
❑ Mindful breathing for 5 minutes

3:30 P.M.
❑ Reward yourself with a massage, seaweed wrap, pedicure, or some other relaxing luxury

6:00 P.M.
Dinner: Mediterranean Lamb Shanks with Kalamata Olives, Capers, and Herbs (page 186)
          Sautéed or steamed spinach (page 177 for basic cooking instructions)

6:45 P.M.
16 ounces filtered water with lemon or lime

7:00 P.M.
❑ Have fun

8:00 P.M.
❑ Sea Salt Glow (page 209), followed by Peppermint and Lavender Foot Soak (page 208) and Revitalizing Foot Scrub (page 208)

9:00 P.M.
❑ Night skin care prescription
  • Cleanser
  • Retinol serum
  • Eye cream
  • Any additional optional age-reducing creams (collagen-producing peptide cream, soy cream, vitamin C cream, etc.)

10:00 P.M. TO 7:00 A.M.
❑ Sleep

STAY YOUNG FOREVER

Congratulations! You have successfully completed the 2-Week-Plan. Not only do you look more youthful and beautiful on the outside, but you also feel more youthful, positive, and energetic on the inside. The changes are so striking that you probably don't need to take a test to see them, but that's what I want you do. To see just how dramatically this program has changed your appearance and your life, I would like you to do the following:

1. Take an "after" photo and compare it to your "before" photo.

2. Place a pH test strip on your tongue and compare it to the results of the strip you used before day 1.

3. Retake the "Test Your Aging Potential" assessment (page 144) and compare your results to the test you took two weeks ago.

The Baby Steps Approach

The vast majority of my patients have used this approach. Instead of tackling all of the Stop Aging Prescription at once, they incorporated just one or two into their lives at a time. Because of this, I can tell you that you will still notice results quickly. I've seen those quick results on the faces of patient after patient after patient.

I recommend you incorporate the Stop Aging prescriptions into your life in this order. Progress through these steps as quickly or as slowly as needed.

Step 1. Make a plan. Read the book and think about the importance of the program. It doesn't matter how long it takes you to complete this step. Don't beat yourself up for your slowness. Feeling guilty or angry at yourself only accelerates aging. So accept yourself as the person you are in this moment, and tackle this step at a pace that works for you. It may take you a few weeks.

To complete your planning:

1. Read the Skin Care Prescription chapter and list the types of products you'll need on a piece of paper. Then turn to the appendix

and pick out brand names that match what you are looking for. Go shopping, either online or in person, and buy what you need.

2. Get the ingredients you'll need to make the Alkalinizing Cocktail. Purchase the greens powder—either Greens First (preferred) or Greens+—the fiber, and any optional ingredients. Purchase your mineral and probiotic supplements as well.

3. Decide what you will do for fun. Read about fun activities in the Lifestyle Prescription chapter.

Step 2. Drink the Alkalinizing Cocktail once or twice a day, increase your consumption of filtered water, and put your fun activity on the calendar.

Step 3. Continue your fun activity (once or twice a week), continue drinking your Alkalinizing Cocktail, continue to increase your water consumption, and start your morning and evening skin care routines.

Step 4. Continue your efforts from step 3 and start taking the rest of your supplements (the mineral supplement with calcium and the probiotic supplement).

Step 5. Overhaul your kitchen. Toss out or give away the sugar, coffee, cola, sweet treats (ice cream, etc.), and alcohol. You may still eat ice cream and other desserts, but only have them away from home. The extra effort required to drive to the local supermarket or ice cream parlor will automatically cause you to indulge less often. Similarly, you may also have wine and other types of alcohol, but you'll drink them a lot less if you don't keep them within easy reach. The same goes for coffee.

Step 6. Stock your kitchen with the Age Stoppers listed in chapter 5. Look over the recipes in this book and plan to make one of those recipes in the near future.

Step 7. Try to increase your consumption of vegetables, aiming for at least 1 cup of greens and 2 cups of vegetables a day.

Step 8. Pick one lifestyle activity (deep breathing, relaxation, etc.) and incorporate it into your life. Once that activity becomes habitual, pick one more, and so on.

Step 9. Make alkalinizing food switches. Using the chart on page 173 as a guide, gradually switch from acid-producing foods and beverages to more alkalinizing foods and beverages. (For more guidance on the pH effects of various foods, see the appendix.)

Make the Alkalinizing Switch

Make these easy switches to improve pH balance. Consult pages 222–225 for a more extensive list of pH values of specific foods.

Switch from this	To this
Table salt	Sea salt
Apple pie	Baked apple
Beans	Lentils
Pale beer	Dark beer
Apple juice	Apple cider
Diner coffee	Organic freshly brewed coffee
Cola	Water with lemon or lime
Rice or soy milk	Almond milk
Black tea	Green or herbal tea
Beef	Organic bison or poultry
Steak and potatoes	Steak strips and vegetable stir-fry
Eggs and bacon	Vegetable omelet with side of fruit
Ham and cheese sandwich	Chef's salad
Bread made from white flour	Bread made from whole-wheat or oat flour
Potato chips and French fries	Sweet Potato chips (page 198)
Candy	Fruit
White rice	Wild rice
Refined pasta	Whole-grain pasta
Butter	Clarified butter (aka ghee)

Step 9 is a continuous, lifelong process. I'm still in step 9—and so are all of my patients. Although you may occasionally take a step back after taking two steps forward, you'll be further along your path to whole-body youthfulness than you were before you started. Keep the focus on what you've achieved and on how great you feel. Nothing is out of your reach!

10

the stop aging recipes

Many of the recipes you'll find showcased in the following pages grew out of a conversation I had with my good friend Greg Thompson, the chef I mentioned earlier. I told him how I had been using a solay—basically water that has been saturated with sea salt—to flavor salads and to marinate meat and fish. "I think you are on to something," he told me after eating a salad flavored with the solay. I was flattered, as Greg knows food and cooking better than anyone I know. *New York Magazine* singled out one of his restaurants for having the "Best Power Lunch in New York."

I gave Greg some sea salt to take with him, and he soon began experimenting at home and in his restaurants. He also soon began sending me various sea-salt-inspired recipes to try, and I found them so delicious that I've included them here for you to enjoy as well.

Greg and New York City–based nutrition consultant Leslie Dantchik, M.S., also created many other recipes after I gave them both this challenge: to design delicious, convenient, and alkalinizing recipes that even the most time-starved and culinarily challenged person could make. They didn't let me down. Their recipes will show you how to easily incorporate the alkalinizing Age Stoppers—especially dark leafy greens—into your daily repertoire.

In this chapter you'll also find a number of "recipes" for your skin. From body scrubs to foot soaks to deodorizing powders, these make-at-home products smell as fantastic as they will make your skin look.

Equipment You Will Need

To make the Stop Aging recipes, you need only a few kitchen basics: a large chef's knife, a wok, a cutting board, and various sizes of saucepans, skillets, and mixing bowls. If you plan to make any of the juice recipes (they are optional), you'll need a good juicer, too. For taste, I recommend you grind sea salt and peppercorns from mills rather than using previously ground pepper or sea salt. For convenience, I suggest you purchase a slow cooker and a cheap spray bottle. Use the bottle to spray solay onto salads, cooked vegetables, and other foods.

Keep solay on hand. To make it, you'll need sea salt crystals, a glass jar with a lid, and filtered water. My favorite sea salt brand for taste and purity is Himalayan Crystal Salt, available online at www.natural-salt-lamps.com/edible-crystal-salts.html. At this site you can purchase glass jars, sea salt crystals, sea salt grinders, and coarse sea salt (among many other sea salt supplies). To make the solay for the first time, place a large salt crystal (it looks like a pink rock) in your glass jar. Fill the jar with water, cover, and let sit for twenty-four hours. The salt will dissolve until it saturates the water. Use as needed, removing the amount of solay you need for a given recipe and then adding more water to replace what you took from the jar. Once the salt crystal fully dissolves, replace it with another crystal.

Cooking Basics

You will use the following cooking and preparation techniques when making Stop Aging recipes:

Blanching. Put 1 pound leafy vegetables into a wire basket, coarse mesh bag, or perforated metal strainer and lower into 2 gallons of boiling water (or use 1 gallon for ½ pound of greens). Cover and cook 2 to 3 minutes. Remove the greens and cool them immediately in ice water for 2 to 3 minutes.

Garlic mashing. Place a peeled garlic clove on a cutting board. Cover the clove with the side of a chef's knife. Carefully push down on the side of the knife blade with your fist to mash the clove. Then mince or chop as directed.

Lemon squeezing. Many of the recipes call for lemon or lime juice. You *could,* for convenience's sake, purchase a bottle of juice at the store. For a better-tasting recipe, however, I recommend you squeeze the juice from real lemons and limes. To easily squeeze a lemon or lime without a mess or having to worry about picking out the seeds, Leslie offers this advice: roll the fruit between palm and counter first, for more juice, then cut the lemon in half and pierce the rind with a fork. Squeeze the lemon rind side down into your dish; half a lemon or lime roughly yields 2 tablespoons (1 ounce) of juice.

Sweating. Garlic and onions are not only alkalinizing but also wonderfully delicious, as long as you don't burn them. To sweat them, coat them with oil (by stirring them in an oil-coated pan and adding oil as needed) and stir over low heat until soft but not brown.

Steaming. In a shallow microwave-safe baking dish, add enough water to cover the bottom of the dish, vegetables, and sliced lemon on top. Cover with a paper towel. Microwave for 3 to 4 minutes, until desired tenderness. The cooking time will depend on the type of vegetable. To quickly flavor any steamed vegetable, spray lightly with solay and serve.

Breakfast Recipes

Although the following recipes may call for some unusual ingredients (I'm willing to bet you've never made eggs with kale before), I'm confident that you'll be quite surprised by their wonderful taste. Healthful eating really can taste wonderful; taste it to believe it.

Blueberry and Sunflower Seed Muffins with Flax

Most muffins are filled with refined sugar and fat and have absolutely no nutritive value whatsoever. The typical mega-muffin sold at your local coffeehouse will set you back about 600 calories—

most of which comes from acid-producing sugar. The following fiber-rich muffin, however, uses oat flour, flaxseed meal, cinnamon, blueberries, and sunflower seeds to alkalinize this traditionally acid-producing breakfast option. (Note: Keep flaxseed meal refrigerated to avoid rancidity.)

This recipe calls for unrefined sugar, made from pressing sugar cane stalks. Muscovado Turbinado and other unrefined sugars contain more molassis—and minerals—than refined sugar, making them less acid producing.

1½ cups oat flour	½ teaspoon sea salt
1 cup flaxseed meal	1 teaspoon cinnamon
½ cup whole-wheat flour	1 cup low-fat milk
1 cup unrefined sugar	2 eggs
2 teaspoons baking soda	1 cup dried blueberries
1 teaspoon baking powder	1 cup sunflower seeds

Mix the first eight ingredients in a large bowl. Stir in the milk and eggs until mixture is smooth. Add the blueberries and sunflower seeds. Mix just enough to combine. Portion into 8 muffin cups. Bake at 375°F for about 15 minutes, until a toothpick inserted in the center comes out clean.
Serves 8

Chai Tea Smoothie with Toasted Coconut and Banana

Most commercial smoothies contain some fruit and a lot of sugar in the form of high-fructose corn syrup. This smoothie recipe, on the other hand, will alkalinize your body with banana and coconut. The chai tea mix lends a decadent flavor that will have you swearing you're drinking a dessert for breakfast.

½ cup flaked coconut, toasted	1 banana
1 cup liquid chai tea mix	1 cup ice

Use unsweetened coconut flakes. Place coconut flakes on a flat pan or cookie sheet and bake at 350°F until golden brown. Set a pinch of coconut flakes aside. Place the chai mix, the banana, the

rest of the coconut flakes, and ice in your blender. Blend until smooth. Sprinkle the remaining coconut flakes on top.
Serves 1

Omelet with Kale, Feta, and Yellow Tomatoes

Many people automatically use spinach in their omelets, so I challenged Greg to create an omelet that featured kale, which is the most alkalinizing green on the planet. He delivered beautifully. Note that this omelet recipe calls for whole eggs rather than egg whites. That's because your skin will benefit from the essential fatty acids, vitamin A, and lecithin in the yolk.

1 tablespoon extra-virgin olive oil	Freshly ground black pepper
½ cup kale, blanched (see page 176)	2 eggs (or 4 ounces pasteurized whole eggs)
2 tablespoons chopped yellow tomatoes	1 tablespoon crumbled feta cheese
Sea salt	1 teaspoon chopped scallions

Heat oil in a nonstick sauté pan over medium heat. Add the kale and tomatoes. Season with the salt and pepper. Stir until tomatoes begin to soften. Add the eggs and cook until they are almost completely cooked through. Add the feta. When the feta begins to melt, fold the omelet in half and slide out onto a plate. Sprinkle scallions on top and serve.
Serves 1

Super Omega-3 Banana Pecan Pancakes with Honey Butter and Maple Syrup

The sugar and refined flour of traditional pancakes leave you feeling drowsy and muddled, not to mention full of acid. This recipe alters this usually empty-calorie dish by adding alkalinizing flaxseed meal, pecans, and banana. To bump up the fiber content of your pancakes, start with a whole-grain mix or recipe made with whole-grain flour. Note that this recipe calls for clarified butter (ghee), usually sold in health food stores or in the ethnic section of the grocery store. If you can't find it, you can make your own by melting unsalted butter over low heat. Once the butter separates, skim off the white foam. Turn off the heat and let sit until the butter stops bubbling. Strain it through a fine sieve or a cheesecloth-lined strainer. The golden yellow liquid you collect is the clarified butter (butterfat). As it cools it will solidify. Cover and store for up to several months in the refrigerator. If you prefer to use a premade mix, simply omit any fat or oil suggested on the mix directions, and instead add 1½ cups of flaxseed meal for every ½ cup of fat. Then follow the recipe directions from "set aside a few banana slices."

1 teaspoon honey	½ teaspoon salt
3 tablespoons butter, softened	1 cup milk
1½ cups flour	2 eggs
1 cup plus 2 tablespoons flaxseed meal	½ banana, thinly sliced
3 tablespoons unrefined sugar	½ cup chopped pecans
1½ teaspoons baking powder	1 teaspoon clarified butter (ghee)
	Maple syrup

Mix 1 teaspoon honey with the 3 tablespoons softened butter. Form by ½ teaspoonfuls into balls and refrigerate.

Combine the flour, flaxseed meal, sugar, baking powder, and salt in a bowl. In a separate bowl, whisk together the milk and eggs. Pour the wet ingredients over the dry ingredients and mix just until combined. Set aside a few banana slices, then add the remaining banana slices and the pecans to the batter and stir just until combined.

Heat a skillet or griddle over medium heat and melt the clarified butter. Spoon ⅓ cup of batter for each pancake onto the griddle. Cook until the top of each pancake is bubbly and the edges look dry. Turn and cook until the bottom is lightly browned.

For each serving, place two pancakes on a plate. Top with 1 ball of honey butter, 2 tablespoons warmed maple syrup, and a few of the reserved banana slices.

Yield: About 6 servings

Vanilla Mango Yogurt Smoothie

If you like mango, you'll love this mango smoothie, made more alkaline thanks to the addition of ground flaxseed. Use an organic yogurt (such as Stoneyfield French Vanilla) to ensure that synthetic hormones and antibiotics stay out of your smoothie. If you would like to further alkalinize the smoothie, consider using plain, unflavored yogurt.

2 cups nonfat or lowfat vanilla or plain yogurt

1 fresh mango, peeled and cubed

1 tablespoon ground flaxseed meal or flaxseed oil

1 teaspoon honey (optional)

1 cup ice

Combine all ingredients in a blender and puree until smooth.
Serves 2 to 4

Greek-Style Yogurt with Grapes, Granola, and Blueberries

The fiber in this seemingly decadent breakfast option will improve digestion. The recipe calls for Greek yogurt (such as Fage brand) because it tends to be thicker and creamier. If you cannot find Greek yogurt, any regular organic brand of sugar-free yogurt will work.

2 tablespoons unsweetened granola

8 ounces nonfat or low-fat Greek yogurt

8 to 10 seedless green grapes

¼ cup fresh or frozen blueberries (thawed if frozen)

1 teaspoon honey (optional)

Reserve a pinch of the granola. Place the rest of the granola and all other ingredients in a medium bowl. Stir until well combined. Sprinkle the remaining granola on top.
Serves 1

Main Courses

You'll find many different salads in the upcoming pages. Use dark leafy greens (instead of iceberg lettuce) as the base of any salad. The darker the lettuce leaf, the more healthful chlorophyll it contains.

To make salad preparation quick and easy, I recommend cooking boneless, skinless chicken breasts ahead of time. They will keep two to three days in the refrigerator. For tender, juicy chicken, try poaching. Bring to a boil enough chicken broth to cover the chicken. For more flavorful chicken, add chopped onion, garlic, carrot, celery, and sea salt to the broth. Reduce the heat, add the chicken, and simmer just until it cooks through, about fifteen to twenty minutes. Alternatively, you can brush the breasts with lemon juice and olive oil and then grill over an open flame until cooked through, about 10 minutes. Finally, you can also roast the chicken in the oven at 425°F for 15 minutes. For all methods, the chicken is done when it reaches an internal temperature of 165°F.

Avocado, Alfalfa Sprout, and Grilled Vegetable Sandwich

You can quickly assemble this incredibly alkalinizing sandwich at home or on the go. If ordering from a deli, choose whatever variety of whole-grain bread is available.

Mustard	½ to 1 cup alfalfa sprouts
2 slices oat bran bread	1 cup grilled sliced vegetables

Spread mustard on the bread. Place the sprouts and veggies between the slices.
Serves 1

Beef Sirloin Stew with Parsnips

This stick-to-your-ribs stew will keep your skin glowing thanks to the carrots, parsnips, and potatoes.

1 pound beef sirloin, in 1-inch cubes	1 large sweet Vidalia onion, in ½-inch dice pieces
Sea salt	2 cups peeled, sliced carrots
1 tablespoon fresh thyme	2 cups peeled, sliced parsnips
Freshly ground black pepper	8 cups vegetable stock
Flour for dredging	2 cups peeled, cubed potatoes
1 cup olive oil	

Season the beef cubes with the thyme. Add salt and pepper to taste. Dredge the seasoned beef in flour. Place a large stock pot over medium-high heat. Add the olive oil and heat until almost smoking. Add the beef cubes and sear until browned. Add the onions, carrots, and parsnips. Cook 5 to 10 minutes or until slightly caramelized and browned. Add the stock, bring to a boil, then immediately reduce heat to a simmer. Cook until the beef is fork tender, about 2 to 3 hours. Add the potatoes and cook 30 minutes longer. Adjust seasoning before serving.

Serves 4

Broiled Scallops

The spices, lemon juice, and olive oil in this recipe help to balance the acid-producing nature of the scallops. Pair it with a vegetable and a salad and you've got a convenient pH-balanced meal.

1 pound bay scallops or sea scallops (halved if using sea scallops)
Sea salt solay (see page 176)
2 tablespoons olive oil
Juice of half a lemon
Freshly ground black pepper
1 tablespoon chopped fresh basil or flat-leaf parsley (optional)

Preheat the broiler. Lightly coat a baking dish with cooking spray. Lightly spray scallops with solay and then season them with olive oil, lemon juice, pepper, and basil or parsley. Place in the baking dish and broil until scallops are opaque, about 3 minutes.

Serves 4

Chopped Tofu Salad

You can probably find many of the ingredients for this recipe at your local supermarket's salad bar. Make sure to chop the lettuce with a knife rather than ripping it.

2 cups chopped lettuce (such as field greens, romaine, or spinach)
Unlimited vegetables of your choice (such as tomatoes, cucumber, mushrooms, onions, broccoli), chopped

½ cup cubed firm, baked or
   steamed tofu
1 teaspoon sunflower seeds
2 tablespoons cooked or
   canned chickpeas

3 tablespoons Alkalinizing
   Salad Dressing (page 200)

Combine all ingredients in a bowl and toss.
Serves 1

Citrus Salmon Salad

Nearly all canned salmon is wild. That's both convenient and beneficial, as farmed salmon may contain PCBs from the fish food. Feel
free to experiment with the amounts of the various recipe ingredients. The greens, veggies, and citrus fruit are all alkalinizing. You
can't overdo them.

Unlimited greens of your
   choice
Unlimited vegetables of
   your choice
One 1.3-ounce can wild
   salmon, drained, rinsed,
   bones removed

Orange slices
Grapefruit slices
Olive oil
Vinegar
Sea salt
Freshly ground black pepper

Mix the greens, vegetables, salmon, orange, and grapefruit. Dress
to taste with olive oil and vinegar, sea salt and pepper.
Serves 1

Curried Chicken Salad with Grapes and Macadamia Nuts

The curry powder, celery, grapes, lettuce, and nuts help to alkalinize the chicken and mayo in this traditional lunch dish.

1 pound diced cooked
   chicken (see page 182 for
   basic chicken cooking
   tips)

1 cup reduced-fat mayonnaise
1 teaspoon curry powder
½ cup finely diced celery

½ cup seedless grapes, halved (or substitute raisins)

¼ cup macadamia nuts, chopped

Red leaf lettuce

Placc all ingredients except the lettuce in a bowl and stir until combined. Chill and serve over the lettuce.

Chicken wrap: Place the chicken salad mixture in a whole-wheat wrap along with lettuce and chopped vegetables of your choice.

Celery snack: Omit the lettuce and instead spread the chicken salad mixture onto celery sticks or endive.

Hors d'oeuvres: Omit the lettuce and instead hollow out plum tomatoes and stuff them with the chicken mixture.

Serves 4 as a main course

Lentil Soup

Lentils are full of fiber, making them great for digestion. They also are highly alkalinizing. For convenience, make this soup ahead of time, storing it in the refrigerator for 3 to 4 days or in the freezer for 2 to 3 months.

1 tablespoon extra-virgin olive oil

1 cup diced sweet onion

1 tablespoon minced garlic

½ cup diced celery

½ cup peeled and diced carrot

Sea salt

Freshly ground black pepper

1 pound lentils

8 cups vegetable broth

½ cup plum tomatoes, roughly chopped

Fresh herbs to garnish

Heat the olive oil in a stock pot over medium-high heat. Add the onions, garlic, celery, and carrots. Season with salt and pepper. Cook until just starting to brown. Add the lentils and stir to combine with other ingredients. Add the vegetable broth and stir. Bring to a boil. Reduce heat to a simmer. Add the tomatoes and let simmer until lentils are soft and cooked completely. Garnish with herbs before serving.

Serves 6 to 8; 1 serving = 1 cup

Mediterranean Crab Salad

The following recipe is designed to be eaten over lettuce, but you may find you enjoy it just as much over tomatoes. Instead of crabmeat, you can also make this salad with any white fish, shrimp, or lobster.

1 cup cooked crabmeat	Sea salt
1 tablespoon lemon juice	Freshly cracked black pepper
1 tablespoon thinly sliced fresh basil	Extra-virgin olive oil
	Lettuce leaves
1 tablespoon chopped flat-leaf parsley	

Combine all ingredients except lettuce in a bowl and adjust the seasoning. Serve over lettuce leaves.
Serves 4

Mediterranean Lamb Shanks with Kalamata Olives, Capers, and Herbs

The variety of spices in this recipe do more than add flavor. They also help to buffer the acids in the lamb.

3 lamb shanks (about 1½ pounds each)	4 large anchovies
Sea salt	8 cups vegetable stock
Freshly cracked black pepper	1 cup kalamata olives
½ cup olive oil	½ cup large capers
2 cups chopped canned or fresh tomatoes	1 teaspoon fresh rosemary
	1 teaspoon fresh thyme
	1 tablespoon fresh basil

Season the lamb with salt and pepper. Heat the oil in a stock pot over medium-high heat. Add the lamb and sear until browned on all sides. Add the tomatoes and anchovies. Reduce heat to medium and cook, stirring occasionally, until the anchovies dissolve, about 3 minutes. Add the vegetable stock, olives, and capers. Simmer

until the lamb is fork-tender, approximately 2 to 3 hours. Add rosemary, thyme, and basil just before serving.
Serves 4

Pepper-Seared Yellowtail Tuna over Salad

All meat produces acid in the body, and tuna is no exception. In this recipe, you counteract the acid-producing nature of the tuna with lots of arugula (a dark leafy green), red onion, sea salt, and the Alkalinizing Salad Dressing.

6 ounces arugula
¼ cup thinly sliced red
   onion
1 small yellow tomato, in
   ½-inch dice
4 tablespoons Alkalinizing
   Salad Dressing (page 200)

8 ounces sushi-grade
   yellowtail tuna, roughly
   1 inch thick
Sea salt
Freshly cracked black pepper
1 teaspoon extra-virgin olive
   oil

Combine the arugula, onion, and tomato. Toss lightly with the salad dressing. Arrange on two plates. Set aside.

Sprinkle the tuna lightly with salt and pepper. Heat the olive oil in a nonstick sauté pan over medium-high heat. Sear the tuna 1 to 2 minutes on each side, just until the fish is golden brown on the outside and rare to medium-rare on the inside. Slice thinly. Place tuna over the salad.
Serves 2

Potato Leek Soup

This recipe works great with Yukon Gold potatoes, which have a lot of flavor and color.

1 tablespoon extra-virgin
   olive oil
2 cups washed, sliced leeks,
   white parts only

1 teaspoon fresh thyme
2 pounds potatoes, peeled
   and sliced 1 inch thick
4 cups vegetable broth

Sea salt

1 tablespoon chopped

Freshly ground black pepper   scallions

Heat olive oil in a stock pot over medium-high heat. Add the leeks and cook, stirring, until soft but not brown. Add the thyme, potatoes, and vegetable broth. Bring to a boil, then reduce heat to a simmer and cook until potatoes are completely soft. Puree with an immersion blender. Season with salt and pepper and garnish with the scallions.

Serves 6 to 8; 1 serving = 1 cup

Sautéed Eggplant in Spicy Tomato Sauce

Serve this vegetable-rich hearty sauce over any high-fiber, whole-grain pasta (see page 221 for recommended brands)

$2\frac{1}{2}$ cups eggplant in
   $\frac{1}{4}$-inch cubes

Sea salt

4 tablespoons olive oil

1 medium onion, chopped

2 cloves garlic, minced

1 teaspoon dried or
   2 teaspoons fresh oregano

1 teaspoon dried or
   2 teaspoons fresh basil

1 28-ounce can crushed
   tomatoes

1 teaspoon crushed red
   pepper flakes (or to taste)

Freshly ground black pepper

$\frac{1}{2}$ pound whole-grain pasta,
   cooked

Grated Parmigiano-Reggiano
   cheese

Sprinkle eggplant with salt and set aside.

Heat 2 tablespoons of olive oil in a medium saucepan. Add onion and cook until translucent, about 10 minutes. Add garlic in the last minute, being careful not to brown it. Add oregano and basil and cook for 30 seconds. Add crushed tomatoes and stir. Add red pepper flakes, salt, and pepper to taste. Continue to cook over low to medium heat, stirring occasionally, for about 15 minutes.

While the sauce is cooking, rinse eggplant and pat dry. Heat remaining 2 tablespoons oil in a nonstick pan. Add the eggplant and turn to coat evenly. Cook until evenly browned and soft. Season with salt and pepper.

Combine the eggplant with the sauce. Reduce heat to a simmer and adjust seasonings. (Note: add $\frac{1}{2}$ cup water if sauce reduces too much.) Serve over pasta, topped with cheese.

Variation: Add $\frac{1}{4}$ cup nonfat or lowfat ricotta cheese.
Serves 4

Sesame-Grilled Chicken Sandwiches with Miso Mayonnaise and Cucumber Slaw

The lime juice, miso, and cucumbers help to alkalinize this delicious recipe. If you are pressed for time, use the precooked chicken that you keep in your refrigerator just for these rushed occasions.

1 pound skinless, boneless
   chicken breasts
$\frac{1}{4}$ cup plus 1 tablespoon
   sesame oil
4 tablespoons lime juice
   (from about 2 limes)

1 tablespoon miso
1 cup reduced-fat mayonnaise
3 large cucumbers, shredded
   on a mandoline or with a
   box grater
8 slices whole-grain bread

Place the chicken, $\frac{1}{4}$ cup sesame oil, and 2 tablespoons lime juice in a zip-top bag. Refrigerate for at least $\frac{1}{2}$ hour and as long as overnight.

Mix the miso with the mayonnaise in a small bowl. Place in the refrigerator until you are ready to use it. Then make the slaw by tossing the shredded cucumber, 2 tablespoons lime juice, and 1 tablespoon sesame oil in a small bowl.

Grill the chicken over an open flame or in a grill pan on the stove until cooked through, about 10 minutes. Slice the chicken.

For each sandwich, place $\frac{1}{4}$ of the chicken, mayo, and slaw between 2 slices of bread.
Serves 4

Seared Tuna

Unlike some other types of fish, tuna tastes best when rare or dark pink in the middle. If you cook it through, it will become too dry.

For this reason, you'll use sushi grade tuna, which is safe to eat rare, for this recipe.

1 tablespoon olive oil	1 tablespoon sesame oil
4 ounces sushi-grade tuna steak	Sea salt
	Freshly ground black pepper

Heat the oil in a nonstick pan over medium-high heat. Brush the tuna with sesame oil and season on both sides with salt and pepper. Add fish to the pan and sear 2 to 3 minutes on each side until golden on the outside but rare in the middle.
Serves 1

Shrimp Garden Wrap

The lettuce, tomato, and onion in this wrap help to counterbalance the acid-producing nature of the shrimp. Use precooked, peeled shrimp to speed up your prep time.

One 6-inch whole-grain, spinach or sun-dried tomato tortilla	4 cooked, peeled, large shrimp, tails removed
Mustard	Chopped lettuce
1 tablespoon reduced-fat mayonnaise	Chopped tomato
	Chopped onion

Spread the tortilla with mustard to taste and the mayonnaise. Place the shrimp on the tortilla, top with lettuce, tomato, and onion to taste, and fold over.
Serves 1

Sliced Turkey Crunch Sandwich

This simple sandwich is brought to life with the addition of thinly sliced apples, which also help to alkalinize this traditionally acid-producing lunch option.

1 Granny Smith apple,
   peeled, cored, and thinly
   sliced
1 tablespoon lemon juice
4 ounces thinly sliced turkey
One hero-style roll
   (whole-grain if possible)

2 tablespoons reduced-fat
   mayonnaise
Sea salt
   Freshly cracked black pepper
3 leaves romaine lettuce

Toss the apple slices with the lemon juice to prevent browning. Discard any extra lemon juice. Place the turkey on the bread. Spread the mayonnaise on top of the turkey. Season with salt and pepper. Top with the apples and the lettuce.

Serves 1

Tricolor Green Salad with Tuscan-Style Strip Steak

In this recipe, the alkalinizing effects of the arugula and other lettuce varieties along with the lemon juice in the dressing offset the acid-producing effects of the steak. For crisper salad greens, soak them in ice water and then thoroughly spin or pat dry.

1 pound strip steak
$\frac{1}{2}$ cup sesame oil
$\frac{1}{4}$ cup lime juice
1 cup baby arugula
1 cup torn radicchio
1 cup torn red leaf lettuce

1 teaspoon lemon juice
1 tablespoon extra-virgin
   olive oil
1 tomato, sliced
$\frac{1}{2}$ red onion, sliced very thin
Balsamic vinegar

Marinate the steak in the sesame oil and lime juice for 1 hour.

Meanwhile, toss the arugula, radicchio, lettuce, lemon juice, and olive oil.

Sear or grill the marinated steak over medium-high heat until it reaches the desired doneness. Remove from the heat and set aside to cool for 10 to 15 minutes, then slice the steak as thinly possible against the grain.

Divide the greens among four plates and ring the salad with the sliced steak. Garnish with the tomato and onion. Drizzle with a splash of balsamic vinegar.

Variation: Instead of the lemon juice and olive oil, use Alkalinizing Dressing (page 200), or simply spray the salad with sea salt solay mixed with a squeeze of lemon.

Serves 4

Tuna with Jicama, Cilantro, and Lime

Jicama is a Central American root vegetable that can be eaten raw. It offers a wonderfully alkalinizing crunch to just about any dish and is a great snack alternative. This salad can be served over lettuce or on whole-grain bread.

8 ounces water-packed
  chunk light tuna
1/2 cup peeled, diced jicama
1 tablespoon chopped
  cilantro
2 tablespoons lime juice

1/4 cup finely diced red onion
1/4 cup finely diced tomatoes
1 tablespoon extra-virgin
  olive oil
Sea salt
Freshly ground black pepper

Combine all ingredients in a bowl and mix well.

Serves 2

White Bean and Chicken Chili

This fiber-rich recipe improves digestion while it alkalinizes. It features the herb cilantro (also called fresh coriander). This herb quickly loses its aroma when heated, which is why you reserve half of it to use as a garnish just before serving.

1 pound chicken breast,
  cut into 1/2-inch cubes
Sea salt
Freshly ground black pepper
1/2 cup olive oil
1 cup diced onion

1 cup diced celery
1 tablespoon minced garlic
1 cup chopped cilantro
4 cups chicken stock
2 cups canned white beans,
  drained and rinsed

Season the chicken with salt and pepper. Heat the olive oil in a stockpot over medium-high heat. Add the chicken, onion, celery, garlic, and half the cilantro. Cook until the chicken is just beginning to brown. Add the stock and bring to a boil. Reduce heat to a simmer and cook until the chicken is tender. Add the white beans and when they are heated, add the remainder of the cilantro and serve. *Serves 4*

Side Dishes

Greens rank as the number one Age Stopper, yet most of us have a very narrow knowledge of greens. Other than the lettuce on our salad and spinach, most of us—myself included—don't know how to prepare greens. Thanks to Chef Greg and Leslie, however, none of us has a good excuse for skimping anymore. In addition to greens, you'll also find a few other very alkalinizing but seldom used side dish ingredients.

Asian Jicama Slaw

Stop Aging eating doesn't get any easier than this no-fuss recipe. It's a wonderful option for a potluck picnic.

2 cups peeled, julienned jicama	1 medium red onion, thinly sliced
1 cup julienned yellow bell pepper	$\frac{1}{2}$ cup lime juice
1 cup julienned red bell pepper	$\frac{1}{4}$ cup sesame oil
$\frac{1}{2}$ cup chopped cilantro	Sea salt
	Fresh cracked black pepper

Combine all ingredients in a bowl. Chill before serving.
Serves 2

Basic Cabbage

Cabbage makes a wonderfully alkalinizing accompaniment for any kind of simply prepared fish or meat. You can make this dish with any type of cabbage—red, green, savoy, bok choy, or Napa. Just vary the liquid you use by the type of cabbage—for example, beer for green cabbage, cider for red cabbage, and soy sauce with sesame oil for bok choy.

¼ cup olive oil	Up to 2 cups beer, cider, or low-
1 large onion, thinly sliced	sodium soy sauce/sesame oil
1 cup cabbage, thinly sliced	mixed with water (¼ cup
	sauce/¼ cup water)

Heat the olive oil over medium-high heat. Add onion and cook until soft. Reduce heat to medium. Add cabbage and cook until soft. Add the liquid and simmer until the liquid is reduced by half.
Serves 1

Braised Red Cabbage: This amazing recipe incorporates six of the Age Stoppers—cabbage, olive oil, onion, apple, apple cider, and sea salt.

¼ cup olive oil	1 small head (1 pound) red
1 large yellow onion, sliced	cabbage, sliced thinly
thinly	2 cups apple cider
2 Granny Smith apples,	Sea salt
peeled, cored, and diced	Freshly ground white pepper

Heat olive oil in a saucepan over medium-high heat. Add the onion and cook, stirring, until soft but not brown. Add the apples and brown lightly. Stir in the red cabbage. Add the cider and reduce heat to a simmer. Cook until cabbage is soft and the cider is mostly reduced. Season with salt and pepper to taste.
Serves 4

Bok Choy and Mixed Vegetables: This cabbage is milder in taste than other cabbage varieties. If you are a cabbage newbie, try bok choy first, as it offers a gentle introduction to this family of greens.

¼ cup peanut oil	1 tablespoon chopped scallions
1 tablespoon minced garlic	1 large head bok choy, sliced
1 tablespoon minced ginger	thinly

Any amount of additional chopped vegetables of your choice (Chinese broccoli, water chestnuts, bell peppers, shiitake mushrooms, snow peas, baby corn, carrots)

½ cup low-sodium soy sauce
1 tablespoon sesame oil
2 tablespoons chopped cashews

In a wok heat oil over high heat. Stir-fry garlic, ginger, and scallions for 30 seconds. Add bok choy and other vegetables and stir-fry until tender-crisp. Be careful not to let the garlic, ginger, and scallions brown. Add soy sauce and sesame oil. Garnish with chopped cashews.

Shrimp, Bok Choy, and Mixed Vegetables: Clean, shell, and devein 20 to 24 large shrimp (about 1 pound). Steam the shrimp until pink. Combine with the bok choy and vegetable mixture and serve.
Serves 4

Basic Greens

You can use this basic recipe to make any type of greens. (Note: blanch kale, broccoli rabe, or green beans before sautéing—see page 176.)

¼ cup extra-virgin olive oil
1 cup pre-blanched greens or 4 cups raw greens
1 tablespoon minced garlic

Sea salt
Freshly ground black, white, or mixed peppercorns
Pinch of red pepper (optional)

Heat oil over medium-high. Add the greens, garlic, salt and pepper, and red pepper. Sauté until tender. Softer greens such as spinach and arugula take only a few seconds to cook. Firmer greens such as escarole, cabbage, and Swiss chard take longer to soften; for these chewier greens, add ½ cup of chicken or vegetable broth to the sauté pan, simmering the greens in the broth until the liquid has reduced by half.

Beans and Greens: Add canned white beans or chickpeas, rinsed and drained.

Whole-Grain Pasta and Greens: Cook $^1\!/_2$ pound whole-grain fenne or linguini. Toss the pasta with the cooked greens.
Serves 4

Kale with Garlic and White Beans

Have you thought about eating more kale but didn't know how to prepare it? This recipe provides the quick, easy, and delicious answer.

1 tablespoon extra-virgin olive oil	One $15^1\!/_2$-ounce can white beans, drained and rinsed
2 tablespoons minced garlic	Sea salt
1 pound kale, blanched	Freshly ground white pepper
1 cup vegetable broth	Grated Parmigiano-Reggiano cheese

Heat the olive oil in a large saucepan over medium-high heat. Add garlic and cook, stirring, for a few seconds. Add the kale and sauté for about 5 minutes until warm. Add the broth and simmer for 10 minutes. Stir in the white beans. Add salt and white pepper to taste and sprinkle with cheese.
Serves 4

Mixed Green Salad

Having a salad at lunch and/or dinner—either as a side or as the main course—is a great way to increase your consumption of the top two Age Stoppers: greens and vegetables. Keep salads interesting by trying different types of greens (mesclun, romaine, arugula, and so on) and vegetables (bell pepper, cucumber, broccoli, cauliflower, carrots, etc.). For an extra alkalinizing zip, add sliced citrus fruit, avocado, apple, or raisins. Add sliced jicama or seeds for extra crunch.

Unlimited salad greens of your choice	Sliced citrus fruit, seeds, jicama, avocado, nuts (optional)
Unlimited chopped or sliced vegetables of your choice	Alkalinizing Salad Dressing (page 200)

Fill a plate with salad greens, vegetables, and any of the optional ingredients you are using. Dress with Alkalinizing Salad Dressing (page 200).
Serves 1

Pureed Butternut Squash

This alkalinizing winter squash is rich in fiber, vitamin C, magnesium, and potassium. Cinnamon further alkalinizes this simple dish.

2 cups peeled, cubed butternut squash	1 tablespoon light butter $1/2$ teaspoon cinnamon

Place squash in a microwave-safe bowl. Add enough water to cover the squash halfway. Cover with a paper towel and microwave on high until the squash is soft, about 4 to 5 minutes. Drain the squash and transfer it to a food processor. Add butter and cinnamon and puree until smooth.
Serves 2

Roasted Brussels Sprouts

If you've shunned Brussels sprouts since childhood, it's probably because you are sensitive to bitter tastes. This cooking method will reduce the bitterness without sacrificing the alkalinizing nature of this wonder food. The sea salt will further suppress your perception of its bitterness.

1 pound Brussels sprouts,
    ends trimmed and cut in
    half lengthwise
2 tablespoons extra-virgin
    olive oil
	2 tablespoons balsamic vinegar
	Sea salt
	Freshly ground black pepper

Preheat oven to 400°. Toss Brussels sprouts with olive oil, balsamic vinegar, salt, and pepper. Coat a baking dish with cooking spray and place Brussels sprouts in the dish. Place the dish on the

top rack in the oven. Bake 30–40 minutes, turning once, until tender and slightly crispy on the outside.
Serves 4

Roasted Tomatoes

This side dish tastes gourmet but takes only a few minutes to prepare and fewer than 10 minutes to cook. It also tastes delicious.

1 pint cherry or grape tomatoes	Sea salt
1 to 2 tablespoons olive oil	Freshly ground black pepper

Preheat the oven to 425°. Coat a shallow baking dish with cooking spray. Gently toss the tomatoes with the oil and season with salt and pepper. Bake until the tomatoes begin to soften and wrinkle, about 8 to 10 minutes.
Serves 4

Sweet Potato Chips

If you love french fries, you'll love this more alkaline version that is packed with beta-carotene to improve skin health.

1–2 medium sweet potatoes, sliced ¼-inch-thick	1 clove garlic, minced
2 tablespoons olive oil	Sea salt
	Freshly ground black pepper

Preheat oven to 350°. Toss the potatoes with the oil, garlic, and salt and pepper. Coat a baking sheet with cooking spray. Arrange the sweet potatoes in a single layer on the baking sheet. Bake for 8 to 10 minutes, checking occasionally to make sure the potatoes do not burn. Flip the potatoes and bake for another 4 to 5 minutes, or until easily pierced with a fork.

Cheese Sweet Potato Chips: Add 1–2 tablespoons freshly grated Parmigiano-Reggiano cheese to the oil you toss the potatoes in.
Serves 2–4

Quinoa Salad

Quinoa is wonderfully alkalinizing, but few people make it because it's not as familiar to us as rice or wheat. This recipe will help you get better acquainted with this ancient South American grain.

4 cups cooked quinoa, cooked following package directions and cooled	½ cup chopped flat-leaf parsley
	¼ cup lemon juice
	¾ cup olive oil
1 cup diced tomatoes	1 medium red onion, diced
½ cup diced red pepper	Sea salt
½ cup diced green pepper	Freshly ground black pepper

Quinoa is easy to cook. Rinse it a few times, drain, and then cook 1 cup quinoa in 2 cups water with 1 teaspoon of salt for 15–20 minutes. Toss the cooked quinoa in a bowl with all other ingredients. Adjust the seasoning to taste. Serve chilled.

Variation: This recipes also tastes fantastic with wild rice, couscous, or barley.

Serves 4

Wild Rice

Follow the package instructions if you have a box of wild rice. I've included this convenient recipe in the event you purchase wild rice in bulk and it comes without cooking instructions.

3 cups water or stock	Sea salt, pinch
1 cup wild rice	

Bring water or stock to a boil and add wild rice. Return to a boil and then reduce heat to a simmer. Cover and cook 40 to 50 minutes, until rice is tender. Drain excess liquid, fluff with a fork, and serve.

Serves 2

Marinades and Dressings

Use the following dressings and marinades to further alkalinize any dish.

Alkalinizing Salad Dressing

Keep a shaker bottle full of this simple dressing on hand at all times. Use it on salads, greens, and literally anything that needs a little extra flavor. I also like to keep a mixture of solay and lemon juice in a spray bottle (the kind hairdressers use to wet hair). I keep it on my table and whenever I'm having salads or greens, I give them a quick spray for extra, alkalinizing flavor.

½ cup sea salt solay (see page 176)

1 tablespoon lemon juice

½ teaspoon freshly cracked black pepper

1 teaspoon chopped flat-leaf parsley

1 tablespoon extra-virgin olive oil

Combine all ingredients in a shaker bottle.
Serves 5–10

Basic Chicken or Meat Marinade

This marinade works great for grilling over a BBQ, as well as for broiled, baked, or sautéed meat or chicken.

1 tablespoon minced garlic

2 tablespoons extra-virgin olive oil

1 tablespoon lemon juice

1 teaspoon sea salt

½ teaspoon freshly cracked black pepper

1 teaspoon chopped flat-leaf parsley

1 teaspoon fresh rosemary leaves

Mix all ingredients. Pour over meat or chicken, cover, and marinate for at least an hour and as long as overnight in the refrigerator.
Makes enough for 1 pound meat or chicken

Basic Fish Marinade

This fish marinade works great for grilling over a BBQ, but the fish also tastes delicious broiled, baked, or sautéed.

1 teaspoon sea salt	1 teaspoon chopped flat-leaf
½ teaspoon fresh cracked	parsley
white pepper	2 tablespoons extra virgin olive oil

Mix all ingredients. Pour over fish, cover, and marinate for at least an hour in the refrigerator.
Makes enough for 1 pound fish

Desserts

By nature, most desserts are sweet, and that sweetness usually comes from a very popular Age Accelerator—sugar. You can reduce some of the acid-producing punch of your dessert by using a more alkaline base of fruit, particularly apples. Experiment with your personal baking recipes and see if you can reduce the amount of added sugar. You may be able to reduce the amount of sugar in a recipe by as much as half and not miss it at all.

Keep in mind that dessert is meant to be enjoyed. Don't drive yourself crazy trying to create 100 percent alkaline desserts. Just enjoy them in moderation and make more alkaline choices whenever possible by adding raisins and oatmeal to cookies, cinnamon to puddings, and fruit juices in place of sugar. The following recipes taste delicious but also offer a nice alkalinizing end to your meal.

Baked Apple

Apples are low-calorie, low-fat, and available year round. The following varieties bake well: Rome, Mutsu, Gala, Jonagold, Granny Smith, and Golden Delicious.

1 apple	¼ teaspoon cinnamon
½ cup 100% cranberry	½ cup low-fat vanilla ice
juice	cream or frozen yogurt
¼ teaspoon nutmeg	1 tablespoon sliced almonds

Preheat the oven to 350°. Slice the apple in half and core it. Pour the cranberry juice in the bottom of a small baking dish. Add the apple to the dish and sprinkle each half with nutmeg and cinnamon. Cover and bake for 20 minutes. Uncover and bake another 10 minutes or until slightly brown. Serve warm with the ice cream and sprinkled with almonds.

Variation: For a sweeter, crunchier treat, add 1 teaspoon unsweetened granola and ½ teaspoon honey at the time you add the spices.
Serves 2

Belgian Waffles

The alkalinizing nature of the banana, strawberries, flaxseed, and spices helps to balance the acid-producing sugars in the yogurt and waffle. You may use any whole-grain waffle for this recipe. I've suggested the Kashi brand because it lends a sweet vanilla flavor to the dessert.

2 Kashi frozen waffles, toasted	½ cup sliced strawberries
	1 banana, sliced
4 ounces vanilla yogurt or Cool Whip topping	1 tablespoon ground flaxseed
	Cinnamon or pumpkin pie spice

Spread the waffles with yogurt. Top with strawberries and banana. Sprinkle with the flaxseed and spice. For a large dessert, serve one waffle per person. For smaller finger-food portions, quarter the waffles before serving.
Serves 2 to 8

Frozen Grapes

Grapes contain enough of the minerals manganese, potassium, calcium, and iron to counterbalance their sugar, making them a wonderfully sweet yet alkalinizing treat. Grapes are also a rich source of the vitamins C and K and a variety of antioxidants, including youth-promoting resveratrol.

1 bunch red grapes, stems removed

Place grapes in a zip-top bag, seal, and freeze overnight.
Serves 4

Crunchy Oatmeal Raisin Cookies with Flax

The flaxseed meal, sea salt, oats, and raisins help to alkalinize these traditionally acid-producing treats.

2 tablespoons unsalted butter, softened	$\frac{1}{2}$ teaspoon sea salt
$\frac{1}{2}$ cup brown sugar	$\frac{1}{4}$ teaspoon baking soda
3 tablespoons flaxseed meal	2 cups steel-cut oats
$\frac{1}{2}$ cup honey	1 cup raisins
1 egg	1 cup chocolate chips, chopped dates, figs, or
$\frac{1}{2}$ cup flour	pecans, in any combination

Preheat oven to 350°F. Cream butter, sugar, and flax meal using the paddle attachment on an electric mixer. Add the honey and egg and mix well. Slowly add in the flour, salt, baking soda, and oats. Stir in the raisins and chips, fruit, or nuts. Shape tablespoonfuls of dough into balls. Bake on a greased cookie sheet for about 15 minutes, until firm.
Makes 2 dozen cookies; 1 serving = 1 cookie

Warm Sliced Apples

This sweet treat is completely pH-balanced. You have nothing to feel guilty about! It's great with low-fat ice cream or frozen yogurt, or as a topping to a slice of angel food cake.

8 apples, peeled, cored, and sliced into eighths	1 stick cinnamon, broken into pieces
$\frac{1}{4}$ cup 100% apple or cranberry juice	$\frac{1}{2}$ teaspoon ground ginger
1 teaspoon ground cinnamon	$\frac{1}{4}$ teaspoon cardamom
	1 tablespoon vanilla
	$\frac{1}{4}$ cup maple syrup

Place apple slices in a large pot. Add cranberry juice and cook over low heat, stirring occasionally to prevent the apples from sticking or burning. As the apples begin to release their own juices, bring to a slight boil. Add ground cinnamon, cinnamon stick, ginger, cardamom, vanilla, and maple syrup. Stir mixture until the apples are evenly coated. Cover and cook at a simmer for about 15 minutes, stirring occasionally, until apples are soft and break easily with a fork.

Almond Apple Slices: Add toasted sliced almonds just before serving for extra crunch and alkalinizing nutrition.

Raisin or Cranberry Apple Slices: Add ½ cup raisins or cranberries to the mixture while cooking.

Serves 4

Juice Recipes

If you're a busy person like me, then I strongly recommend you purchase a juicer and get in the habit of making your own fresh fruit and vegetable juices. The Stop Aging recipes will help you to increase your consumption of fruits and vegetables, but we all have those days when we're go-go-go from morning until night, days when lots of chopping seems overly time-consuming. Your juicer beautifully does the prep for you. If you buy a good one, you can stick just about anything in it without having to worry about it clogging or breaking. In my experience, paying $100 more for a better-quality juicer is well worth it. The better juicers can manage anything you give them. They also last longer and come with excellent warranties.

Fresh fruit and vegetable juices are rich in vitamins, minerals, and enzymes. They are the best vitamin and mineral supplements around—fresh from your fridge. Below you will find my favorite recipes.

Apple Ginger Fizz

1 inch ginger	1 apple, cored
2 or 3 carrots	Shot of seltzer water

Place first three ingredients in juicer. Pour in a glass and mix with seltzer.

Serves 1

Alkalinizing Punch

3 kale leaves

2 or 3 carrots

1 apple, cored

Wedge of lime or lemon

Place first three ingredients in the juicer. Pour in a glass, add a squeeze of lime or lemon, and stir.

Serves 1

Cleansing Cocktail

2 or 3 carrots

1 apple, cored

$\frac{1}{2}$ beet

Three kale leaves

1 inch ginger

Place all ingredients in the juicer. If desired, mix with crushed ice.

Serves 1

Pineapple Punch

2 or 3 slices fresh
   pineapple

$\frac{1}{2}$ cucumber

1 apple, cored

Place ingredients in juicer.

Serves 1

Breakfast Juice

3 or 4 slices pineapple

1 apple, cored

4 or 5 strawberries

Place ingredients in juicer.

Serves 1

Skin Care Recipes

The recipes you'll find in this section are for your skin, not your stomach. Your skin will absorb the ingredients in your soaks and scrubs, which is why I've chosen naturally detoxifying ingredients such as sea salt and specific oils. The essential oils in these recipes are concentrated—a tiny bit goes a very long way. Going beyond the two to four drops I recommend in each recipe can easily create an irritating and overpowering scrub.

You may add fresh fruit to any scrub recipe. My favorites are papaya and pineapple because they contain exfoliating enzymes. Avocado is also a great choice because it is extremely emollient.

If you choose to make larger amounts at one time, store the excess in the refrigerator in a wide-topped glass jar with a tightly fitting lid.

Calming Lavender Rose Sugar Scrub

1 cup granulated cane sugar	1 teaspoon evening primrose oil
¼ cup of almond or grape seed oil	2 to 4 drops lavender essential oil
	2 to 4 drops rose essential oil

Combine sugar, almond or grape seed oil, and evening primrose oil. Blend well until mixture has a paste-like consistency. Add essential oils and blend well. Massage onto wet skin and rinse.
Makes enough for more than one application. Store extra scrub in the refrigerator.

Deodorizing Powder

To keep your body smelling spring fresh despite less frequent showering, try this make-at-home powder. Choose either bergamot, cinnamon, or lavender essential oil, as all three offer natural antibacterial properties.

¼ cup cornstarch	3 to 5 drops essential oil
¼ cup baking soda	(bergamot, cinnamon, or lavender)

Combine cornstarch and baking soda. Add essential oil and blend well. Sprinkle powder on clean, dry skin.
Makes enough for more than one application

Eye Puffiness Home Remedy #1

Caffeinated tea bags contain tannins and natural astringent properties that soothe away puffiness. Herbal chamomile tea bags contain the puffiness reducer bisabolol.

2 tea bags, black or chamomile

Steep teabags in boiling water for 10 to 15 minutes. Remove from water and place in the refrigerator until cool. You may either place the cool teabags directly on your lids or saturate cotton balls with tea and place them on your eyes.
Yields 1 application

Eye Puffiness Home Remedy #2

Potatoes contain the enzyme catecholase, which also acts as a skin lightener.

1 baking potato

Cut the potato into thin slices. Place slices into cool water to keep them crisp and prevent browning. When you're ready, place cool slices directly over eyes. Store excess potato in cold water in the refrigerator.
Yields 1 application

Papaya Walnut Sea Salt Scrub

A friend, Mary McGuire, a natural foods expert, created this recipe. You may substitute chopped almonds for the walnuts.

¼ papaya
1½ cups sea salt
¼ cup chopped walnuts
¼ cup almond or olive oil

1 or 2 drops orange essential oil
1 or 2 drops vanilla essential oil or 1 teaspoon vanilla extract

Cut papaya in half and remove seeds. Scoop papaya into bowl and mash well. In a separate bowl, combine salt and walnuts. Add the almond or olive oil to the salt and nut mixture, blending until sticky. Add papaya and mix well with a wooden spoon, forming a uniform, thick paste. Add orange essential oil, then vanilla essential oil or extract. Mix thoroughly. Massage onto wet skin and rinse.

Peppermint and Lavender Foot Soak

½ cup Epsom salts	3 drops peppermint essential oil
½ cup sea salt	3 drops lavender essential oil

Add Epsom salts and sea salt to 1 gallon warm water. Set aside for 10 minutes, until dissolved. Stir in peppermint and lavender oils. Soak feet 10 to 15 minutes. Follow with the Revitalizing Foot Scrub. *Yields 1 soak*

Revitalizing Foot Scrub

1½ cups sea salt	2 to 4 drops lavender essential oil
⅓ cup avocado or sweet almond oil	2 drops peppermint essential oil

Combine sea salt and avocado or almond oil by gradually adding oil to sea salts and mixing well. Add essential oils and mix until combined.

Use after the Revitalizing Foot Soak. Massage over your feet, paying special attention to heels and soles. Rinse and follow with a thick, rich moisturizer.

Makes enough for more than one application. Store excess in the refrigerator.

Revitalizing Sea Salt and Sugar Body Scrub

½ cup granulated sugar	2 to 4 drops grapefruit essential oil
½ cup sea salt	2 to 4 drops orange essential oil
¼ cup grape seed oil	
2 teaspoons evening primrose oil	

Combine sea salt and sugar and blend well. Add grape seed oil and evening primrose oil, blending into a paste. Add orange and grape-fruit essential oils. Massage onto wet skin and rinse.

Makes enough for more than one application. Store excess in the refrigerator.

Sea Salt Glow

This is a fantastic at-home detoxification treatment that leaves the skin wonderfully soft. Put it on your skin before relaxing with pota-toes or tea bags on your eyes or before relaxing in a foot soak, for a complete at-home spa experience.

½ cup fine sea salt (or whirl coarser salt in a food processor)

1 cup sweet almond, avocado, apricot kernel, jojoba, or olive oil

2 tablespoons evening primrose oil (optional)

4 drops lavender essential oil

Combine all ingredients and mix well. After your shower, slowly massage mixture in a circular motion all over clean, damp skin. Wait 20 minutes and then rinse in lukewarm water.

Makes enough for more than one application. Store excess in the refrigerator.

11

stop aging for life

Are you amazed by how far you have come? In just two weeks you have transformed your appearance, health, and life. Every cell in your body can now communicate easily with all the others, forming the connections needed to power your body and mind with optimal energy. You are in charge of your health, career, relationships, and beauty. You smile naturally because you are happy. You are confident, energetic, and calm. You are beautiful on the inside and out!

Let's keep you this way. Right about now you may worry—as I did after my first juice fast—that you'll never be able to keep this up, that you'll eventually backslide and end up looking and feeling the way you did two weeks ago. Well, you know what? That isn't going to happen. First, feeling and looking good is contagious. Now that you feel fantastic, you have the energy and motivation you need to stay that way. Second, the more alkaline you become, the more your tastes change. You'll come to prefer Stop Aging eating and come to hate how cruddy you feel after eating acid-producing foods. Finally, I'm going to teach you, throughout the pages of this parting chapter, how to maintain your momentum.

Maintaining your results requires a balance of perseverance—following your Stop Aging Prescriptions as closely as possible—and realism. This is life, after all, and the rest of your life will be filled with change—in the form of travel, career moves, family challenges, relocations, you name it. From time to time your life will become incredibly busy. When this happens, you might find that you skip some of the Lifestyle Prescriptions, stop eating your greens (because you never got to the grocery store to buy them), and fall into bed at night without doing your skin care routine. You will not always be perfect, but I am willing to put money on the fact that you will continually maintain some aspects of the program at all times. No matter what is going on in your life, you will be better off than you were before day 1.

No matter how far you backslide, you'll eventually look in the mirror and notice that you don't look as good as you once did. You'll notice you don't have as much pep as you used to, and you will say to yourself, "Aha—I need to start doing *x, y,* and *z* again." When this happens, help yourself to get back on track by using the Stop Aging Daily Organizer in the appendix (page 225). It provides you with a to-do list you can copy and use daily to ensure you complete all of your Stop Aging tasks. Also, try to solve the problems that caused you to stray. This will help you to more firmly recommit yourself, so the next time you won't stray quite so far.

How do I know that this will work? I know because my life is anything but predictable. As I was writing this book, I experienced many life challenges. My children, both teenagers, tested me on many occasions. My husband and I didn't always agree on the best way to handle our rebellious children, which at times created tension between us. My father's health was also failing, with him going in and out of the hospital. I also was taking on new responsibilities for my career—writing a regular column for a Web site, putting together this book, and handling interview after interview for the media. It seemed as if my life never stopped, yet I hung on to what I knew was most important. I drank my alkalinizing cocktails religiously, took my supplements, followed a nearly perfect skin care regimen, kept my juicer on my kitchen counter at all times, and did the best I could with my lifestyle and eating.

In the following pages you'll find my advice—gained from my personal experience as well as the experiences of many patients— for remaining pH-balanced during some of the more challenging aspects of the rest of your life.

Let's start with eating out. When life gets busy, most of us head to the nearest restaurant.

The Stop Aging Eating Out Guide

Restaurant eating can be just as alkalinizing as eating at home, if you prepare and make better choices.

Read the menu at home. Many restaurants post their menus on-line. They usually also don't mind faxing or mailing a menu to you or simply telling you the specials over the phone. Make your choice at home, as this will help you stick to it once you are hungry and surrounded by the tempting sights and smells of the restaurant. I know I'm much more likely to order acid-producing foods if I make my choice at the restaurant, especially after a glass of wine has weakened my resolve.

Bank up your alkalinizing calories. Eat healthfully throughout the day, maximizing your alkalinizing food choices. This will create a buffer for any acid-producing foods you eat at the restaurant as well as motivate you to continue to eat healthfully at the restaurant.

Start with the right mind-set. Have an Alkalinizing Cocktail and/or glass of water with lemon before you head out the door. It will take the edge off and put you in a healthful frame of mind. The cocktail will also give you an alkalinizing boost that will counteract any acid-producing foods you eat at the restaurant.

Arrive only slightly hungry, not ravenous. Hunger almost always leads to poor choices. If needed, have a small alkalinizing snack—such as a few raw vegetables—before leaving for the restaurant.

Enjoy every bite. Savor your food, even if you are drinking wine (an Age Accelerator) or eating a steak (another Age Accelerator). Guilt, anxiety, and frustration will only set off the acid-producing stress response. On the other hand, if you delight in every bite, you'll create joy-producing neurochemicals that will add a glow to your skin, even if what you are eating isn't all that good for you.

Eat slowly. Start the meal feeling calm. Before you take your first bite, put down the fork and take a deep breath. Then, as you begin to eat, chew your food thoroughly, until it's well mashed in your mouth. This will improve digestion, especially after eating a so-called recipe-for-indigestion meal. The slower eating pace will also give you time to reevaluate your eating decisions, so that you'll find the motivation to pack up half of that steak or burger in a take-home container.

In the following pages you'll find specific ordering tips for breakfast (especially diner eating) and lunch or dinner.

EATING OUT TIPS FOR BREAKFAST

Choose water with lemon as your beverage. If you'd prefer juice, make sure it's freshly squeezed. Otherwise you'll probably end up with a sugar-added store brand. If you want to sip something hot, opt for green or herbal tea instead of coffee. Diners are notorious for leaving a pot of coffee on a hot burner all day long, and coffee becomes more acidic the longer it sits on a burner. They also make the coffee from grounds that may have been sitting around for weeks or months. Although whole coffee beans will last up to two weeks at room temperature and longer in the refrigerator or freezer, grinding exposes coffee to oxygen, causing it to break down quickly. The shelf life of ground coffee is only a few days, but you can bet it's been sitting around the diner much longer, as most establishments buy coffee in bulk. If you've ever wondered why you get heartburn after drinking diner coffee, now you know why. Instead, treat yourself to freshly ground and brewed coffee from a coffeehouse on the way home.

Now that you know what you will and won't be drinking at the diner, let's talk about what you'll be eating. In general, the following options are best:

• An omelet packed with veggies such as onion, bell pepper, spinach, asparagus, and so on. Pay more for extra veggies if the diner provides only two choices with the omelet. Substitute fruit for the bread or fried potatoes that usually accompany the meal.
• Oatmeal. Order a side of fruit.
• High-fiber breakfast cereal with milk and a side of fruit.

EATING OUT TIPS FOR LUNCH AND DINNER

I eat out a lot, so I can tell you with confidence that the vast majority of restaurants actually do offer many alkalinizing options. The trick is being assertive and asking for substitutions. Restaurants make their living serving patrons and keeping them happy. Most will gladly alter any of their dishes for you.

Try these tips when eating out:

• Get rid of the bread basket or say no to the waiter if he passes it around. Nearly all restaurant bread is made with refined flour, providing you with empty, acidifying calories. If you need to munch while waiting, ask for a plate of vegetables such as celery or carrots.

• As with bread, nearly all restaurants serve pasta made with refined flour. If you need to satisfy a pasta fix, then do so, but choose a smaller pasta appetizer rather than a main course and split it with your dining companions. That way you can indulge in the taste and texture you crave, but hold yourself to a much smaller portion.

• Have a green salad or vegetable-based soup as your appetizer. Top your salad with oil and a squeeze of lemon rather than the dressings offered by the restaurant. Restaurant dressings are often loaded with sugar.

• Swap the grain that comes with the meal (it's almost always refined) with a vegetable such as sautéed spinach or broccoli.

• Get a side of veggies if they don't come with the meal. If the restaurant does not list vegetables as side dish offerings, scan the various main courses and see what vegetables come with them. If you notice that the fish of the day comes with asparagus or the pasta is tossed with broccoli, then you know for a fact that those vegetables are available. Agree to pay extra.

• Ask for a sweet potato instead of white rice or french fries.

• Drink water with lemon, and ask for a few extra lemon wedges—the single one most restaurants provide as a garnish won't squeeze much juice into your water. Or borrow a wedge from one of your dining companions.

• If you order fish, chicken, or beef (or another type of meat), pay attention to the serving size listed on the menu. Order the smallest steak, usually a petite filet mignon. If the size is not listed, ask. This will help you to determine how much to allow yourself (remember to hold yourself to 8 ounces daily). You might bank up for a meal by going vegetarian for breakfast and lunch and carnivorous only at dinner. Remember: if you go overboard, don't feel guilty. Just add an extra scoop of greens powder to your Alkalinizing Cocktail the next morning.

- If you are having pizza, order a thin crust to cut down on acid-producing refined carbs. Top it with lots of veggies, especially onions and garlic.

- Order fruit-based desserts such as chocolate-covered strawberries or apple crisp.

Marcy Gunner Stopped Aging!

"I first saw Dr. Graf very recently for a routine skin check. I chose her mostly because I didn't want to have to stand in my underwear while a male doctor looked me up and down, checking for moles. I found her so lovely and warm that the routine checkup led to me trying her program.

"I had used various skin care products before I met Dr. Graf, but the ones that she suggested to me were more effective. What made the most difference was the Alkalinizing Cocktail. When Dr. Graf first suggested it to me, I thought, 'I don't know how I am going to do this.' I'm up early in the morning and I do enjoy my coffee. But I've found a way to work the cocktail in twice a day, and it's really made a difference.

"My skin looks so much better. I did not look bad before. I never had a lot of blemishes. I did have some wrinkles, yes. Now they are less noticeable, especially the ones on my forehead and around my eyes. It wasn't until someone else mentioned the changes to me that I realized how different I looked. About a month after starting the program, I was sitting around with a bunch of other teachers — all women in their twenties and thirties. We were sitting around talking, and the other teachers began saying to me, 'Wow, you have such good skin. Your skin looks great.' They were right. It does, and I owe it to Dr. Graf."

— MARCY GUNNER,
sixty, kindergarten teacher

The Stop Aging Travel Guide

It was my travel schedule that originally caused me to search for the Alkalinizing Cocktail. I knew I needed to pack something with me that could counteract the acid-producing choices that I sometimes had to make because I honestly had no other option. (Case in point: take a flight that requires a layover in the Detroit airport and let me know if you can find anything alkalinizing to eat.)

Make your Alkalinizing Cocktail your number one travel companion. If you don't have room for the entire container of greens powder, then use a brand such as Greens+, which comes in travel-sized packages, or scoop out the amount you will need into a zip-top bag. You might even create many individual pre-mixed bags of greens powder, fiber, and spirulina (if you use it). Roll them up and place them inside a shaker bottle. Ideally you'll want to keep your greens powder cold, so pack the bottle in an insulated lunch pouch with a cold pack if possible. Once you get to your hotel, store it in the mini refrigerator.

Pack the rest of your supplements either in resealable bags or in a small pill container that you can carry in your purse. Try to pack some healthful snacks for the flight, such as trail mix and/or dried fruit.

Once you arrive at your destination, be religious about your supplements and cocktail. Consider doubling up on Alkalinizing Cocktails while you are gone. Also, use the Stop Aging Eating Out Guide, as you'll be doing a lot of restaurant dining. No matter what, enjoy yourself.

The Stop Aging Party Guide

If you are going to a party, my number one rule is this: enjoy yourself. That's what parties are for. You can take a few steps to alkalinize the experience, but don't let these overshadow your party experience. Parties are all about indulgence, and assuming you go to only a few a year, they won't set you back too much.

That said, you can reduce the acid-producing nature of parties with the following advice:

• Eat your meal at home, planning to just have a few tastes of the party fare.

• Down an Alkalinizing Cocktail before you head out the door. It will help to buffer much of what is to come!

• Alternate every alcoholic drink with a glass of lemon water.

• Choose alkalinizing foods whenever possible. Most party fare includes a plate of raw vegetables and sliced fruit. Stay near those options and away from the little hot dogs wrapped in dough. Once you fill up on fruits and vegetables, leave the scene. If you don't hover near the buffet table, you'll be much less likely to continually pop miniature meatballs and cheese cubes in your mouth.

• Whenever you take a bathroom break, check in with yourself. Close your eyes, focus inward, and take a few deep breaths. Notice your thoughts and emotions. Are you having the time of your life or just killing time? If the latter, consider whether you might have a more productive evening somewhere else. If the former, keep those joyful neurochemicals flowing!

Grow Younger Every Day

One evening while I was watching television, I came across a documentary that featured dozens of vibrant, active men and women in their seventies, eighties, and nineties. They all shared one trait: when asked, "When was the best time of your life?" they all enthusiastically answered, "My best years are right now!" These seniors were making their golden years glitter—and we all have much to learn from them when it comes to skin rejuvenation!

Much like the seniors I just mentioned, I don't talk about "anti-aging" or "turning back the clock." These terms imply that the best part of your appearance—and your life—is over, that you want to present some semblance of your former self. Rather, I'm pro-aging, or supportive of proactive aging. I believe in aging with vitality and vibrancy. I believe that if we all live our lives this way, every day gets better and better.

You are now ready to live your life in this way. You are now ready to live your best years. I'm thrilled you decided to commit yourself to the Stop Aging, Start Living Plan. I hope you are as delighted by your results as the hundreds of patients I've introduced the program to have been over the years. Where do you go from here? Your opportunities are endless. Not only are you looking better, you are living better. You are now ready to take on everything and anything. You are ready to experience joy on a regular basis. You have the energy and confidence to live your best life. Go live it, and enjoy!

appendix

RECOMMENDED PRODUCTS

Greens Powders

Greens First: www.
doctorsfornutrition.com
Greens+: www.greensplus.com

Powdered Fiber Supplements

Benefiber regular or "plus calcium"
powder
Fiber-sure

Probiotic Supplements

Natren: www.natren.com
Allergy Research Group: www.
allergyresearchgroup.com
Metagenics: www.metagenics.com
Pure Encapsulations: www.
purecaps.com
Nature's Way Primadophilus Optima
(sold in stores and online)
Pro-Bio Intestinal Flora Balance—
Microflora Balance: www.
enzymedica.com/products

Mineral Supplements with Calcium

Nature's Plus—Dyno-Mins
Multi-Mineral
Pure Encapsulations—Osteobalance
pH-ion—Alkalive Blue: www.
ph-ion.com
pH-ion—Alklive pH Booster Kit:
www.ph-ion.com

pH Testing Strips

www.ph-ion.com
www.greatestherbsonearth.com
www.vaxa.com
www.indigo.com

Skin Care Products

pH-BALANCED CLEANSERS
Facial Cleansers for All Skin Types
Aveeno Positively Radiant Soap-Free
Cleanser
Cetaphil Soap-Free Cleanser

Facial Cleansers for Oily or
Acne-Prone Skin
Aveeno Clear Complexion Foaming
    Cleanser

Facial Cleansers for Dry Skin
Neutrogena Sensitive Skin Solutions
    Cream Cleanser for Dry Skin
SkinCeuticals Cleansing Cream

DAYTIME MOISTURIZERS
All Skin Types
Aveeno Positively Radiant Daily
    Moisturizer SPF 15 or 30
L'Oreal Anthelios SX with
    Mexoryl SX

For Dry Skin
Eucerin Extra Protection Moisture
    Lotion SPF 30
Jergens Shea Butter Enriching
    Moisturizer

For Adult Acne Prone Skin
Olay Total Effects Daily Moisturizer
    with Salicylic Acid
Aveeno Clear Complexion Daily
    Moisturizer with Total Soy and
    Salicylic Acid
L'Oreal Daily Adult Acne Regimen

NIGHT MOISTURIZERS
Roc Retinol Correxion—Deep Wrin-
    kle Night Cream
Neutrogena Healthy Skin Anti-
    Wrinkle Intensive Serum

Additional (Optional) Age Reducers
L'Oreal Wrinkle De-Crease Night
    Cream
Olay Regenerist Daily Regenerating
    Serum

To Treat Skin Discoloration and
Pigmentation
Neutrogena Visibly Even Night
    Concentrate
Aveeno Postively Radiant

FACIAL SUNBLOCKS (STAND-ALONE)
Aveeno Continuous Protection
    Sunblock—SPF 30 UVA/UVB
Neutrogena Ultra Sheer Dry-Touch
    Sunblock SPF 55 with Helioplex
    UVA/UVB

EYE CREAMS
Olay Regenerist Eye Lifting Serum
Clean & Clear Morning Glow Eye
    Brightening Cream
Roc Retinol Correxion Eye Cream
Neutrogena Radiance Boost Eye
    Cream
Aveeno Positively Radiant Eye
    Brightening Cream

MINERAL MAKEUP
Jane Iredale Mineral Makeup
Neutrogena Mineral Sheers Powder
    Foundation

HOME EXFOLIATION KITS
Neutrogena Advanced Solutions
    Microdermabrasion System
Neutrogena Advanced Solutions
    Facial Peel System
Olay Microdermabrasion and Peel
    System
Olay Thermal Skin Polisher

ACNE TREATMENT PRODUCTS
Neutrogena Advanced Solutions
    Acne Mark Fading Peel
L'Oreal Daily Response—Intensive
    Adult Acne Peel

CLEANSING WIPES
Neutrogena Gentle Makeup Remover
  Pads

BODY LOTIONS AND CREAMS
Cetaphil Cream
Eucerin Cream
CeraVe Cream

NATURAL BODY OILS
Neutrogena Light Sesame Oil
Hermal Body Oil
Alpha-Keri Oil
Robathol

NON-SOAP BODY BARS AND CLEANSING GELS
Aveeno Moisturizing Shower &
  Bath Oil
CeraVe Hydrating Cleanser
Cetaphil Gentle Skin Cleanser
Neutrogena Energizing Sugar Body
  Scrub, Fresh Citrus

HAND CREAM
Neutrogena Norwegian Formula
  Hand Cream
Eucerin Plus Intensive Repair Hand
  Creme

BODY SUNBLOCK—UVA/UVB
Neutrogena Ultra-Sheer Dry-Touch
  Sunblock—SPF 55
Coppertone Spectra 3—SPF 50
Blue Lizard Australian Sun
  Products—SPF 30

BODY SUNBLOCK SPRAYS—UVA/UVB
Coppertone Kids Continuous Spray
  Sunscreen—SPF 50
Neutrogena Fresh Cooling Body Mist
  Sunblock—SPF 30

Aveeno Continuous Protection
  Spray—SPF 30
Banana Boat Spray—SPF 30

Convenient Food Products
HIGH-FIBER BRANDS
Breakfast Cereals
Kellogg's All Bran
General Mills Fiber One
Kashi GoLean (e.g., Good Friends)
Post 100% Bran Cereal
Nature's Path Organic Flax
  Plus Multibran

Pastas
Annie's Homegrown Whole Wheat
Barilla Plus
Heartland Multigrain or Whole
  Grain
Hodgson Mill Whole Wheat Pasta
Mueller's Multigrain

Waffles
Kashi GoLean
Van's
LifeStream Flax Plus

FROZEN FOODS
Ian's baked frozen sweet potato
  fries
Alexia baked frozen sweet potato
  and regular potato fries

SEA SALT
Himalayan Crystal Salt, www.
  natural-salt-lamps.com/
  edible-crystal-salts.html

Juicers
Omega Model 4000 juicer
Champion juicer

PH VALUES OF SELECTED FOODS

Here I've provided you with a rough guide for pH-balanced eating. For a more extensive food-by-food breakdown of hundreds of acid and alkalinizing foods, I highly recommend *The Acid Alkaline Food Guide* (Square One Publishers, 2006) by Susan Brown, Ph.D. I also want to caution you that the effect of food on pH is not an exact science. If you consult many different pH food guides, either in books or on the Internet, you'll uncover some discrepancies. For example, some guides say that spinach is alkalinizing, whereas others say it is acid-producing. Some guides say tomatoes are acid-producing, whereas others say they are alkalinizing. Why the differing results? Food scientists are using differing methods for determining a food's effect on body chemistry. Some foods—such as tomatoes and spinach—are difficult to quantify because they contain natural acids that may or may not be easily metabolized by the body. I've placed many of these debatable foods under the "gray areas" heading.

Finally, pH is just one of many nutritional factors that affect your health. Some very wholesome foods—including some whole grains, vegetables, and fruit—are slightly acid-producing. Because these foods contain high amounts of antioxidants and other nutrients that probably counterbalance any increase in acid, I've listed them under the "gray areas."

Acid-Forming

Alcohol
    Dark beer
    Pale beer*
    Mixed drinks*
    Wine
Animal and fish protein
    Beef*
    Chicken
    Clams
    Fish, all varieties
    Lamb
    Oysters
    Mussels
    Pork
    Scallops
    Shrimp*
    Squid

*Extremely acid-producing

    Turkey
    Venison
Artificial sweeteners
    Aspartame
    Saccharin
Cheese (all varieties)
Cooking oils
    Canola
    Sesame
    Soybean
    Sunflower
Coffee
Eggs
Fast food
    Burgers*
    Burritos*
    Chicken nuggets*
    French fries
    Fried or baked fish
    Fried onion rings

Sandwiches made with meat or
  cheese*
Flour, refined
Ice cream, commercially
  prepared
Milk
  Cow's milk
  Soy milk
Pudding
Refined wheat products
  Bread, white*
  Cake*
  Crackers, saltine*
  Doughnuts*
Rice, white
Salad dressings
  Caesar
  French
  Ranch
  Thousand Island
Salt, table*
Snack foods
  Crackers*
  Cheese puffs
  Pork rinds*
  Potato chips*
  Pretzels*
Soft drinks*
Spreads
  Butter
  Cream cheese
  Jam sweetened with sugar or
    high-fructose corn syrup
  Jelly sweetened with sugar or
    high-fructose corn syrup
  Mayonnaise
  Peanut butter
Sweeteners
  Brown sugar
  Corn syrup
  High-fructose corn syrup
  Stevia

Sugar, white*
Vegetables
  Carrots, non-organic
  Corn
  Peas
White vinegar
Yeast*

Alkalinizing
Bragg Liquid Aminos
Culinary oils
  Flaxseed oil
  Olive oil
Dried fruit
  Raisins
Fast food
  Baked potato with skin
  Fruit bowl
  Hash browns
  Salad
Fruit
  Apples
  Apricots
  Avocado
  Banana
  Blackberries*
  Blueberries
  Cantaloupe*
  Honeydew
  Lemon*
  Lime*
  Mango
  Oranges
  Papaya
  Pineapple
  Raspberries*
  Strawberries*
  Watermelon*
Fruit juices
  Apple

*Highly alkalinizing

Grape

Grapefruit

Orange

Pineapple

Herbs and spices

Black pepper

Cinnamon

Dill

Ginger*

Paprika

Parsley

Scallions

Sea salt*

Miso

Nuts and seeds

Almonds

Cashews

Chestnuts*

Pumpkin seeds*

Sesame seeds

Salad dressings

Alkalinizing Salad Dressing

(page 200)

Olive oil and apple cider vinegar

Spreads

All-fruit, organic

Almond butter

Apple butter

Cashew butter

Ghee (clarified butter)

Sweeteners

Molasses, organic

Rice syrup

Sucanat (evaporated cane juice)

Oats

Oatmeal

Tamari

Tea

Green tea

Herbal tea

Topical oils

Avocado

Coconut

Evening primrose

Flaxseed

Macadamia

Olive

Vegetables

Asparagus*

Beets

Bell peppers

Broccoli

Brussels sprouts

Cabbage

Carrots, organic

Cauliflower

Celery*

Collard greens*

Cucumbers

Dandelion greens*

Kale*

Kohlrabi*

Endive*

Garlic*

Onions

Parsnips*

Potatoes, with the skin

Radishes

Seaweed (nori)

Spirulina

Sprouts (any variety)*

Squash

Sweet potatoes*

Turnips*

Yams*

Zucchini

Vinegar

Apple cider

Umeboshi

Water

Filtered

Mineral*

Purified (bottled)

Gray Areas

These foods are somewhat acid-producing but contain antioxidants and other health-promoting nutrients.

Black tea

Brown rice

Cranberries

Dates

Figs

Honey

Maple syrup

Pomegranates

Rye products

Spinach

Tomatoes

Wheat bran

Whole wheat products

Yogurt (unflavored)

THE STOP AGING DAILY ORGANIZER

Photocopy this chart and use it to stay on track after you finish the Two-Week Plan.

❑ Test saliva pH* _____ (fill in pH value)

❑ Morning skin care routine (cleanser, moisturizer, eye cream, SPF)

❑ Alkalinizing Cocktail

❑ Probiotic supplement

❑ Mineral supplement with calcium[†]

❑ Filtered water (4 liters daily)[††]

❑ Fun activity (1–2 times a week)

❑ Exercise (4 times a week)

❑ Deep breathing (5 minutes, twice a day)

❑ Laughter (1+ daily)

❑ Relaxation (10 minutes, 2 times a day)

❑ Evening skin care routine (cleanser, retinol moisturizer, eye cream, other creams)

❑ Dark leafy greens (1 cup)

❑ Organic vegetables (2 cups)

❑ Fruit (2 servings)[§]

*Eventually your saliva pH should remain between 6.5 and 7.5. The best time to test your pH is about one hour before a meal or two hours after a meal. Test your pH two days a week.

[†]Take at a different time of day than the Alkalinizing Cocktail.

[††]Drink most of your water between meals rather than with meals.

[§]Try to eat fruit as between-meal snacks.

selected bibliography

Chapter 2: The pH Connection

Barzel US, Massey LK. Excess dietary protein can adversely affect bone. *Journal of Nutrition.* 1988;128:1051−3.

Brown S., Jaffe R. Acid-alkaline balance and its effect on bone health. *International Journal of Integrative Medicine.* 2000;2(6):7−15.

Brown, S. Excessive acidity may aggravate urinary disorders. *Total Health.* 2005;25(3):22, 23.

Caso G, Garlick PJ. Control of muscle protein kinetics by acid-base balance. *Current Opinion in Clinical Nutrition and Metabolic Care.* 2005 Jan;8(1):73−76.

Frassetto L, Morris RC Jr., Sellmeyer DE, Todd K, Sebastian A. Diet, evolution and aging—the pathophysiologic effects of the post-agricultural inversion of the potassium-to-sodium and base-to-chloride ratios in the human diet. *European Journal of Nutrition.* 2001 Oct;40(5):200−13.

Gwynn RC, Burnett RT, Thurston GD. A time-series analysis of acidic particulate matter and daily mortality and morbidity in the Buffalo, New York, region. *Environmental Health Perspectives.* 2000 Feb;108(2):125−33.

Hu JF, Zhao XH, Parpia B, Campbell TC. Dietary intakes and urinary excretion of calcium and acids: a cross- sectional study of women in China. *American Journal of Clinical Nutrition.* 1993;58:398−406.

Lemann J Jr., Lennon EJ. Role of diet, gastrointestinal tract, and bone in acid-base homeostasis. *Kidney International* 1972;1:275−79.

Mellen PB, Bleyer AJ, Erlinger TP, Evans GW, Nieto FJ, Wagenknecht LE, Wofford MR, Herrington DM. Serum uric acid predicts incident hypertension in a biethnic cohort: the atherosclerosis risk in communities study. *Hypertension.* 2006 Dec;48(6):1037–42.

Remer T. Influence of nutrition on acid-base balance—metabolic aspects. *European Journal of Nutrition.* 2001 Oct;40(5):214–20.

Sebastian A, Frassetto LA, Sellmeyer DE, Merriam RL, Morris RC Jr. Estimation of the net acid load of the diet of ancestral preagricultural Homo sapiens and their hominid ancestors. *American Journal of Clinical Nutrition.* 2002 Dec;76(6):1308–16.

Taylor EN, Mount DB, Forman JP, Curhan GC. Association of prevalent hypertension with 24-hour urinary excretion of calcium, citrate, and other factors. *American Journal of Kidney Diseases.* 2006 May;47(5):780–89.

Chapter 3: The Digestion Connection

Bezkorovaniny A. Probiotics: determinants of survival and growth in the gut. *American Journal of Clinical Nutrition.* 2001;73(2)Suppl:399S–405S.

Gibson GR. Understanding prebiotics in infant and childhood nutrition. *Journal of Family Health Care.* 2006;16(4):119–22.

Kalliomaki M, Salmininen S, Arvilommi H, Kero P, Koskinen P, Isolauri E. Probiotics in primary prevention of atopic disease: a randomized placebo controlled trial. *Lancet.* 2001;357(9262):1076–9.

Krasse P, Carlsson B, Dahl C, Paulsson A, Nilsson A, Sinkiewicz G. Decreased gum bleeding and reduced gingivitis by the probiotic *Lactobacillus reuteri. Swedish Dental Journal.* 2006;30(2):55–60.

Manning TS, Gibson GR. Microbial-gut interactions in health and disease: Prebiotics. *Best Practice and Research: Clinical Gastroenterology.* 2004 Apr;18(2):287–98.

Moro G, Arslanoglu S, Stahl B, Jelinek J, Wahn U, Boehm G. A mixture of prebiotic oligosaccharides reduces the incidence of atopic dermatitis during the first six months of age. *Archives of Disease in Childhood.* 2006 Oct;91(10):814–9.

Passeron T, Lacour JP, Fontas E, Ortonne JP. Prebiotics and synbiotics: two promising approaches for the treatment of atopic dermatitis in children above 2 years. *Allergy.* 2006 Apr; 61(4):431–37.

Roberfroid MB. Prebiotics and probiotics: are they functional foods? *American Journal of Clinical Nutrition.* 2000;71(6)Suppl:1682S–1687S.

Tuohy KM, Rouzaud GC, Bruck WM, Gibson GR. Modulation of the human gut microflora towards improved health using prebiotics—assessment of efficacy. *Current Pharmaceutical Design.* 2005;11(1):75–90.

Chapter 4: The Joy Connection

Asami DK et al. Comparison of the total phenolic and ascorbic acid content of freeze-dried and air-dried marionberry, strawberry and corn using conventional, organic, and sustainable agricultural practices. *Journal of Agricultural and Food Chemistry.* 2003;51:1237–41.

Bilkis M, Mark K. Mind-body medicine. *Archives of Dermatology.* 1998;134(11):1437–41.

Brandt K, Molgaard JP. Organic agriculture: Does it enhance or reduce the nutritional value of food plants. *Journal of Science in Food and Agriculture.* 2001;81:924–31.

Carbonaro M et al. Modulation of antioxidant compounds in organic vs. conventional fruit (peach, *Prunus persica L.*, and pear, *Pyrus communis L.*). *Journal of Agricultural and Food Chemistry.* 2002;50:5458–62.

Chiu A, Chon S, Kimball A. The response of skin disease to stress. *Archives of Dermatology.* 2003;139:897–900.

Chuh A, Wong W, Zawar V. The skin and the mind. *Australian Family Physician.* 2006 Sep;35(9):723–25.

Fraser GE, Shavik DJ. Ten years of life: Is it a matter of choice? *Archives of Internal Medicine.* 2001;161:1645–52.

Garg A, Chren M, Sands L, Matsui M, Marenus K, Feingold K, Elias P. Implications for the pathogenesis of stress-associated skin disorders. *Archives of Dermatology.* 2001;137:53–59.

Gupta MA, Gupta AK. Psychodermatology: an update. *Journal of the American Academy of Dermatology.* 1996 Jun;34(6):1030–46.

Gupta MA, Gupta AK. Stressful major life events are associated with a higher frequency of cutaneous sensory symptoms: An empirical study of non-clinical subjects. *Journal of the European Academy of Dermatology and Venereology.* 2004 Sep;18(5):560–65.

Havlik RJ, Vukasin AP, Ariyan S. The impact of stress on the clinical presentation of melanoma. *Plastic and Reconstructive Surgery.* 1992 Jul;90(1):57–61.

O'Sullivan R, Lipper G, Lerner E. The neuro-immuno-cutaneous-endocrine network: Relationship of mind and skin. *Archives of Dermatology.* 1998;134(11):1431–35.

Robbins C. *Poisoned Harvest: A Consumer's Guide to Pesticide Use and Abuse.* London: Victor Gollancz.

Saul AN, Oberyszyn TM, Daugherty C, Kusewitt D, Jones S, Jewell S, Malarkey WB, Lehman A, Lemeshow S, Dhabhar FS. Chronic stress and susceptibility to skin cancer. *Journal of the National Cancer Institute.* 2005 Dec 7;97(23):1760–67.

Vena J, Graham S, Hellmann R, Swanson M, Brasure J. Use of electric blankets and risk of postmenopausal breast cancer. *American Journal of Epidemiology.* 1991;134(2):180–85.

Chapter 5: The Stop Aging Nutrition Prescription

Davis P, Polagruto J, Valacchi G, Phung A, Soucek K, Keen C, Gershwin M. Effect of apple extracts on NF-KB Activation in Human Umbilical Vein Endothelial Cells. *Experimental Biology and Medicine.* 2006;231:594–98.

Elsner RJ, Spangler JG. Neurotoxicity of inhaled manganese: Public health danger in the shower? *Medical Hypotheses.* 2005;65(3):607–16.

Cho E, Chen WY, Hunter DJ, Stampfer MJ, Colditz GA, Hankinson SE, Willett WC. Red meat intake and risk of breast cancer among premenopausal women. *Archives of Internal Medicine.* 2006 Nov;166:2253–9.

Huff-Lonergan E, Baas TJ, Malek M, Dekkers JC, Prusa K, Rothschild MF. Correlations among selected pork quality traits. *Journal of Animal Science.* 2002 Mar;80(3):617–27.

Kenefick RW, Hazzard MP, Mahood NV, Castellani JW. Thirst sensations and AVP responses at rest and during exercise-cold exposure. *Medicine and Science in Sports and Exercise.* 2004 Sep;36(9):1528–34.

Lonergan SM, Stalder KJ, Huff-Lonergan E, Knight TJ, Goodwin RN, Prusa KJ, Beitz DC. Influence of lipid content on pork sensory quality within pH classification. *Journal of Animal Science.* 2007 Apr;85(4):1074–9.

Massey, L. Dietary animal and plant protein and human bone health. *Journal of Nutrition.* 2003;133:862S–865S.

Nuckols J, Ashley D, Lyu C, Gordon S, Hinckley A, Singer P. Influence of tap water quality and household water use activities on indoor air and internal dose levels of trihalomethanes. *Environmental Health Perspectives.* 2005;113(7):863–70.

Purba M, Kouris-Blazos A, Wattanapenpaiboon N, Lukito W, Rothenberg E, Steen B, Wahlqvist M. Skin wrinkling: Can food make a difference? *Journal of the American College of Nutrition.* 2001;20(1):71–80.

Reddy ST, Wang CY, Sakhaee K, Brinkley L, Pak CY. Effect of low-carbohydrate high-protein diets on acid-base balance, stone-forming propensity, and calcium metabolism. *American Journal of Kidney Diseases.* 2002 Aug;40(2):265–74.

Rogers EJ, Milhalik S, Orthiz D, Shea TB. Apple juice prevents oxidative stress and impaired cognitive performance caused by genetic and dietary deficiencies in mice. *Journal of Nutrition, Health and Aging.* 2004;8(2):92–97.

Sgan-Cohen HD, Newbrun E, Huber R, Tenebaum G, Sela M. The effect of previous diet on plaque pH response to different foods. *Journal of Dental Research.* 1988 Nov;67:1434–7.

Spangler JG, Elsner R. Commentary on possible manganese toxicity from showering: Response to critique. *Medical Hypotheses.* 2006;66(6):1231–3.

Sponheimer M, Passey BH, de Ruiter DJ, Guatelli-Steinberg D, Cerling TE,

Lee-Thorp JA. Isotopic evidence for dietary variability in the early hominin *Paranthropus robustus*. *Science*. 2006 Nov 10;314(5801):980–82.

Switzer JA, Rajasekharan VV, Boonsalee S, Kulp EA, Bohannan EW. Evidence that monochloramine disinfectant could lead to elevated Pb levels in drinking water. *Environmental Science and Technology*. 2006 May 15;40(10):3384–7.

Tchantchou F, Chan A, Kifle L, Ortiz D, Shea TB. Apple juice concentrate prevents oxidative damage and impaired maze performance in aged mice. *Journal of Alzheimer's Disease*. 2005 Dec;8(3):283–87.

Vijayakumar C, Wolf-Hall CE. Evaluation of household sanitizers for reducing levels of *Escherichia coli* on iceberg lettuce. *Journal of Food Protection*. 2002 Oct;65(10):1646–50.

Winston C. Health promoting properties of common herbs. *American Journal of Clinical Nutrition*. 1999 (Sept);70(3):4915–4995.

Chapter 6: The Stop Aging Supplement Prescription

Annapurna VV, Deosthale YG, Bamji MS. Spirulina as a source of vitamin A. *Plant Foods for Human Nutrition*. 1991;41:125–34.

Chamorro G, Salazar M, Favila L, Bourges H. Pharmacology and toxicology of *Spirulina alga*. *Revista de Investigation Clinica*. 1996;48:389–99.

Gonzalez R, Rodriguez S, Romay C, et al. Anti-inflammatory activity of phycocyanin extract in acetic acid–induced colitis in rats. *Pharmacological Research*. 1999;39:1055–9.

Hayashi O, Hirahashi T, Katoh T, Miyajima H, Hirano T, Okuwaki Y. Class specific influence of dietary *Spirulina platensis* on antibody production in mice. *Journal of Nutritional Science and Vitaminology*. 1998;44(6):841–51.

Thomas D. A study on the mineral depletion of the foods available to us as a nation over the period 1940 to 1991. *Nutrition and Health*. 2003;17:85–115.

Chapter 7: The Stop Aging Skin Care Prescription

Babyak M, Blumenthal J, Herman S, Khatri P, Doraiswamy M, Moore K, Craighead E, Baldewicz T, Krishnan R. Exercise treatment for major depression: Maintenance of therapeutic benefit at 10 months. *Psychosomatic Medicine*. 2000;62:633–38.

Bernardi L, Sleight P, Bandinelli G, Cencetti S, Fattorini L, Wdowczyc-Szulc J, Lagi A. Effect of rosary prayer and yoga mantras on autonomic cardiovascular rhythms: Comparative study. *British Medical Journal*. 2001;323:1446–9.

Michna L, Wagner G, Lou Y, Xie J, Peng Q, Lin Y, Carlson K, Shih W, Conney A, Lu Y. Inhibitory effects of voluntary running wheel exercise on

UVB-induced skin carcinogenesis in SKH-1 mice. *Carcinogenesis*. 2006 Oct;27(10):2108–15.

Schwartz C, Meisenhelder JB, Ma Y, Reed G. Altruistic social interest behaviors are associated with better mental health. *Psychosomatic Medicine*. 2003 Sep-Oct;65(5):778–85.

index

about the author

DR. GRAF is a leading skin-science expert and a board-certified, clinical, and research dermatologist.

Known for her extensive and comprehensive approach to dermatology, Dr. Graf combines minimally invasive office procedures and effective skin care products with fundamental nutrition and lifestyle counseling to elicit both an inner and outer beauty from each of her patients.

Prior to completing her residency in dermatology at the New York University Medical Center, Dr. Graf earned her medical degree from the State University of New York School of Medicine at Buffalo.

Committed to research and the science of natural ingredients from an early point in her career, Dr. Graf was a research fellow and protégé of George Martin, M.D., lab chief and one of the most highly respected scientists in the world, at the National Institutes of Health (NIH).

There, she received an award for Outstanding Achievement from the National Institutes of Health, in addition to obtaining an NIH patent for her research on peptides in 1987. In fact, Dr. Graf is noted for discovering a specific peptide responsible for cell attachment, which was able to inhibit and block melanoma metastases in the lungs of mice.

Today, Dr. Graf continues to research new active ingredients, as well as plant-derived enzymes and peptides, for use in anti-aging products and treatments.

Published in prestigious journals such as the *Journal of Cell Biology* and the *Proceedings of the National Academy of Sciences,* Dr. Graf also wrote the chapter on "Anti-aging Skin Care Ingredient Technologies," which explains the molecular changes at the cellular level and the impact of nutrients on physiological processes, for the dermatology textbook *Cosmetic Dermatology*.

In addition, Dr. Graf is highly regarded as an expert resource and has been quoted in many magazines, including *Allure, InStyle, Prevention, Self, Family Circle, Fitness, Marie Claire, Cosmopolitan, Elle,* and *Essence.* She has also been a guest on television shows such as *The View* and appears regularly on the *Home Shopping Network* with her successful line of dermatology-strength skin care.

Dr. Graf serves as a consultant and advisory board member for a number of cosmetic and pharmaceutical companies, including Johnson & Johnson, Roc, Neutrogena, Medicis, Allergan, and Aveeno. She performed some of the earliest studies on soy technology used in the Aveeno product line and participated in its successful market launch. Dr. Graf also serves on the educational faculty of Allergan and Medicis, where she lectures and teaches other aesthetic physicians how to inject Botox and Restylane.

A member of several professional societies, including the American Academy of Dermatology and Society of Investigative Dermatology, Dr. Graf has lectured nationally and internationally to both dermatologists and plastic surgeons.

She maintains a private practice in Great Neck, New York.